LIVING RIGHT

The Ideal of a Moral-Spiritual Therapy

GENE M. ABROMS, MD

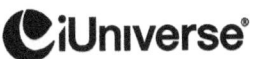

LIVING RIGHT
THE IDEAL OF A MORAL-SPIRITUAL THERAPY

iUniverse books may be ordered through booksellers or by contacting:

iUniverse
1663 Liberty Drive
Bloomington, IN 47403
www.iuniverse.com
1-800-Authors (1-800-288-4677)

ISBN: 978-1-4917-3063-8 (sc)
ISBN: 978-1-4917-3065-2 (hc)
ISBN: 978-1-4917-3064-5 (e)

Library of Congress Control Number: 2014906285

Printed in the United States of America.

iUniverse rev. date: 09/03/2014

Do not imagine that character is determined at birth. We have been given free will. Any person can become as righteous as Moses or as wicked as Jeroboam. We ourselves decide whether to make ourselves learned or ignorant, compassionate or cruel, generous or miserly. No one forces us; no one decides for us, no one drags us along one path or the other. We ourselves, by our own volition, choose our own way . . .

How do we fix these traits into our character? By repeatedly doing them, returning to them until they become second nature.
—Moses Maimonides, twelfth-century physician-philosopher

Precisely as in a dream it is our own will that unconsciously appears as inexorable objective destiny, everything in it proceeding out of ourselves and each of us being the secret theater-manager of our own dreams, so also . . . reality the great dream, that a single essence, the will itself, dreams with us all our fate, may be the product of our inmost selves, of our wills, and we are actually ourselves bringing about what seems to be happening to us.
—Thomas Mann, twentieth-century novelist and essayist

If you know art and science, you already have religion; if you do not, you need religion.
—Goethe, eighteenth-century poet-philosopher

Every one who is seriously involved in the pursuit of science becomes convinced that a spirit is manifest in the laws of the Universe—a spirit vastly superior to that of man . . .
__ Albert Einstein, twentieth-century physicist

CONTENTS

Introduction: The Purpose, Plan and Spirit of the Book...........................ix

Chapter 1:   Beyond Psychology to Spiritual Knowing.............................. 1

Chapter 2:   The Spiritual Framework....................................... 12

Chapter 3:   Personal Dimensions of Spiritual Therapy 35

Chapter 4:   The Will: Its Paralysis and Activation 59

Chapter 5:   The Divided Will 82

Chapter 6:   The Spiritual Group and Outpatient Milieu Therapy 111

Chapter 7:   The Moral Code and the Spiritual Group........................... 134

Chapter 8:   Character Development...168

Chapter 9:   Empathy...190

Chapter 10: The Calling 210

Chapter 11: Blessedness 227

Introduction

THE PURPOSE, PLAN AND SPIRIT OF THE BOOK

In this work I propose a treatment philosophy that goes beyond symptom relief and psychological understanding to achieve moral-spiritual awareness and growth. This heightened awareness gives us values and ideals that are self-evidently and universally true. We can come to know them by transcending ordinary empirical consciousness to achieve a state of intuitive consciousness, a state that, at its fullest development, can give us access to a universal mind-will, which I call Spirit. Accepting the fruits of intuitive awareness fundamentally alters how psychiatry and psychotherapy are conceived and practiced. Therapy ceases to be merely nondirective and relative to individual needs, however respectful and evocative these positions often prove to be, to become a value-guided journey of the soul. Although defining and drawing out the clinical implications of this viewpoint are essential to this work, this is not a clinical manual, much less a work of science or scholarship. It is rather a philosophical treatise with clinical illustrations. It is a practical philosophy of the means required to achieve the ends of freedom of will, authenticity of self, strength of character, and compassionate empathy, among a host of other spiritual ideals.

The framers of the Declaration of Independence affirmed the existence of intuitive moral truth by declaring that "we hold these truths to be self-evident, that all men are created equal, that they are endowed . . . with certain inalienable Rights, that among these are Life, Liberty and the pursuit of Happiness." If these truths are not intuitively self-evident to patients, a therapy grounded in spiritual awareness offers the possibility that they might become so.

I want to show how taking account of the spiritual reality adds another dimension to psychiatric and psychotherapeutic treatment, transforming it from a limited applied science to the expanded scope of a healing art and science. In contrast to those who advocate a spiritual approach at the expense of other dimensions of therapy, I affirm my identity as a physician who has undergone and values psychoanalytic treatment and the results of practicing and teaching the combined medical, psychodynamic, cognitive-behavioral, group, and family therapy approaches. Therefore, engaging with the spiritual reality, rather than diminishing the importance of these other more basic approaches, seeks to build on their capacities to allay symptoms, resolve conflicts, and promote fruitful patterns of working and relating; it seeks to take the further step of promoting the value changes that lead to living a spiritual life.

Promoting value change in patients is a sensitive and painstaking process because it must be done in full awareness of the individual aspirations of the true, authentic self residing within each of us. This respectful awareness limits the work of the spiritual therapist to guiding patients to realize their unique potentials in a spirit of collaboration rather than nondirection, much less imposition.

My journey down this path was initially stimulated by some deeply personal experiences of music, nature, and racial persecution, some of which I shall refer to in subsequent chapters. I owe a great debt to studying the moral philosophies of Immanuel Kant and, in our time, John Rawls and Derek Parfit.[1] I am also indebted to many of my teachers in developing this approach. The staff at the Massachusetts Mental Health Center during my time at Harvard Medical School (1955-1959) left an indelible imprint. Some of these refugees from Nazi-devastated Europe had direct connections to Freud's inner circle. The certainty with which they propounded their idealistic theories, of all places in the land of William James's pragmatism, yielded the intellectual indigestion that typically accompanies severe cognitive dissonance.

Many of my classmates gave up on Freudian theory altogether. How could such seemingly profound insights depend so heavily on personality theories with only tenuous connections to observable facts? How could Bach's vast creative output be construed not as the manifestations of a distinct creative force, but as mere products of sexual sublimation? Did Bach not also father twenty children in addition to all his cantatas, concertos, and masses? Such a concept, a "sublimation" that keeps giving without taking anything away from basic drives, is surely a concept that takes away more than it gives. Better to admit the existence of a wider array of irreducible aspirations and driving forces than those derivable from the sexual and aggressive instincts. These include strivings for competence, mastery, meaning, creative expression, healing, self-actualization, altruism, and loving-kindness—in essence the whole array of spiritual ideals that Abraham Maslow called "being needs."[2]

Yet I ultimately came to appreciate Freud's creative genius in deriving an intellectually challenging philosophy of life from his clinical practice and the philosophy of science of his era. Over time it also became apparent to me that his notion of the unconscious repressed provided a pathway to the conception of a spiritual unconscious. And I was moved by his emissary teachers for their spiritual devotion to patients, which made it possible for us students to listen to the bizarre, disturbing outpourings of fellow damaged souls with a measure of compassion. Some of these teachers had already begun to integrate psychodynamic understanding with the larger body of neuropsychiatric knowledge and humanistic values, pointing the way to the integrative thinking for which we students greatly hungered at the time and continue to do so.

An awe-inspiring teacher at Harvard, Elvin Semrad, demonstrated the intuitive leaps that make it possible to directly know other peoples' private thoughts, feelings, and fantasies. Later when I taught at the University of Wisconsin, my colleague Carl Whittaker also possessed this gift in abundance, which he demonstrated on a regular basis when we worked as co-therapists with staff groups and families. We might walk into a room to see a family for the first time, and Whittaker would immediately point out who was the favorite child or who was having an incestuous relationship and then ask other family members, seemingly out of the blue, what impact these facts were having on their lives. I had a burning desire to find out how Semrad and Whittaker, and later the hypnotherapist Milton Erickson,[3] performed their "magical" feats of intuition and healing. Their insights and maneuvers came so naturally to them that they showed little inclination to grapple seriously with how they had come by their knowledge. What theories they did propose were often tangential, if not entirely irrelevant, to the magnitude of their gifts.

The Plan of the Book

The first chapter describes a series of coincidences that led me into the fields of psychiatry and psychotherapy and that seemed to guide my fledgling attempts at clinical practice. I discuss the crucial differences between the scientific-empirical and the moral-spiritual conceptions of knowledge. In the second chapter, I elaborate on the argument for adding the spiritual dimension to psychotherapy by distinguishing between neutral, objective treatment and inspirational healing that takes advantage of patients' faith and utilizes the so-called placebo effect to maximum extent. In the third chapter, I go into more detail about what I mean by "spiritual" and what is involved in a spiritual therapy. I place great emphasis on intuition and moral and aesthetic experience as ways of gaining access to spiritual knowledge. I assume that our main purpose in life is to discover and realize its ultimate meaning, which is the actualization of the higher self—the "god" or "better angels"—lying within us. We do this through locating our core, true self and following its guiding spirit to realize our will to love, health, and truth. The ultimate fulfillment of this task is to discover our calling and a state of blessedness wherein we achieve communion or "oneness" with all-awareness, with the world soul, with Spirit.

The subject of the purpose of life—of living right—runs throughout the book and comes in for final consideration in the last two chapters (chapters 10 and 11). In the intervening chapters, I discuss the role of depression in paralyzing the will and the role of medication and psychotherapy in freeing the will to find a calling that mends and weaves the fabric of a world and that offers grace and blessedness in return (chapter 4).

I give special consideration to the role of dissociative splitting in compromising the freedom of the will. The result of splitting is the formation of an internal saboteur that typically works against the aims of the true self but sometimes preserves its integrity by thwarting the most ill-conceived plans of a false self (chapter 5).

In this work, I am very preoccupied with the spiritual potential of properly managed groups. Although I recognize that groups structured to maximize spiritual intensity can miscarry and become fanatical cults, I propose a set of rules that, when properly applied, provide a bulwark against this disastrous outcome. Many readers will be surprised to learn that these rules do not prohibit outside socializing among group members. In fact, I contend that outside socializing is a valuable adjunct to generating the shared knowledge and emotional intensity that spiritualizes a group. But the terms of this socializing must be strictly defined and monitored (chapter 6).

In chapter 7, I discuss the relevance of the spiritual group to gaining the intuitive awareness and critical thinking that gives us access to a universal moral code and the means of resolving moral conflicts and dilemmas. Without strong character, one may know the good intellectually without being able to do the good. The group will can sometimes add the character strength to make this possible. The necessity and methods of character development are the subjects of chapter 8. Along with intuition, compassionate empathy, or the capacity to put oneself caringly in others' shoes, is vitally necessary to doing right by them—that is, to do what is interpersonally and socially good (chapter 9).

The Spirit of the Book

This is a positive, optimistic book about our spiritual potential.[4] It focuses more on how we can transcend the past to become richly spiritual rather than be bound by it to suffer exile, like a modern Philoctetes, on a bare island of missed opportunities, past regrets, and festering wounds. Where there is living spirit, civilization has no insuperable discontents, no losses that cannot be risen above.[5] To connect to Spirit is to be inspired to transcendence.

I have tried to write this book in a nontechnical language that is readily accessible and meaningful to clinical practitioners of psychiatry and psychotherapy and their students. It is meant for aspiring professionals to whom a spiritual approach to therapy and life is welcome but in need of clarification. It is offered in the spirit that much work still remains to be done for psychotherapy and human beings to reach their spiritual potential, a potential that comes ever closer to fulfillment when we gain the capacity to enlarge and transcend the personal self, to move toward identifying with and uniting with the higher, universal Self, whose substance is permeated with value—good on balance yet with a dark side. This identification can be achieved through first coming to know what lies in the depths of our own soul and in the souls of loved ones, who thereby constitute with us a unified whole. This knowledge leads us arduously but inevitably to contribute to the world's blessings and to fight its miscarriages. Socrates said, "To know the good is to do the good," provided, of course, that intuition is clear and character is strong. We might also add that to truly know evil, the ever-present underside of the good, is to fight unceasingly to overcome it.

Chapter 1
BEYOND PSYCHOLOGY TO SPIRITUAL KNOWING

Summary. I describe how a guiding hand in the person of an Air Force colonel led me into the field of psychiatry after a false start in surgery. From the beginning, surprisingly good results accompanied my efforts to practice psychiatry. Patients' strong will to health proved to be an essential prerequisite to these results. But serendipity and synchronicity also appear to play a large role in the would-be spiritual therapist's efforts to relieve patients of their psychiatric maladies. Here I offer a preliminary account of the contrasts between the limited perspective of scientific empiricism and the inclusive scope of spiritual knowing.

In 1960, I reported to an Air Force base in New Mexico to serve a two-year term as a flight surgeon. I had just finished my surgical internship, which proved to be a terrible mismatch of my abilities and true interests and the program's requirements. I was now trying to figure out what kind of medical career I was best suited for. As my wife and I were having lunch at the base officers' club, the hospital commander came in to greet us. After the usual pleasantries, he announced, "Abroms, you are our new base psychiatrist." Surprised, I asked how he had arrived at this decision. Pointing to my folder, he replied, "I see here that you went to Harvard and majored in philosophy." Although for form's sake I challenged his paralogic, the truth was that his conclusion seemed right. I had had a go at psychotherapy during college and had gone to medical school with the intention of becoming a psychiatrist. But my psychiatry rotations had been disappointing, whereas surgery, at the dawn of heart operations, was very seductive. So here I was a failed surgeon about to become base psychiatrist with no training and possibly no talent for the work. But as it turned out, the hospital chief's proposal was a godsend. In no time at all, I found myself intensely engaged with patients and on the way to finding not only a profession but a calling.

The first patient I encountered as base psychiatrist was brought to the emergency room in a comatose state by her jet mechanic husband. I had a hunch that the coma was hysterical, which I tested out by pressing my knuckles forcefully into her sternum. (The surgeon mindset dies a slow death). Confirming my suspicion, she promptly woke up and made an office appointment for the next day. After I reviewed her medical and psychological history and confirmed that her coma was in fact a conversion symptom of thwarted anger, she proceeded to analyze herself with no apparent help from me. Over the next six sessions this high school graduate reviewed her childhood disappointments, her struggles with her mother, her sibling rivalries, her transference of feelings onto her husband, and the frequent psychosomatic crises that resulted from trying to manage her painful feelings. She hardly let me get a word in edgewise during this surprisingly sensitive and self-aware recital, some of which resembled my own past history and the issues of my prior therapy. After the sixth session, she stood up, pronounced herself cured, and thanked me profusely for my help. I protested, "Wait a minute—I haven't even started yet!" She was shocked and not a little hurt by my reaction. As time passed, I came to a better understanding of what had transpired between us.

Some fifteen years later, now a formally trained clinician and teacher of psychiatry in a medical school, I was referred a very attractive college freshman, who was manifesting symptoms of anorexia nervosa. Jane had been a prom queen in her senior year at high school but since starting college had lost twenty pounds to reach the mid-nineties, which at a height of 5'7" made her look rail thin. She subsisted on lettuce, low-calorie dressing, and many cans of diet cola, all in an effort to deal with imagined obesity. By the time she reached eighty-five pounds, Jane felt too weak to carry books to class, and she was showing typical symptoms of depression.

Since she continued to lose weight despite my concerted efforts, I called an emergency family meeting, necessitating a long trip by her parents from western Pennsylvania to Philadelphia. I found out during the conference that Jane's eating disorder symptoms of bulimia and anorexia, followed by cessation of menstruation, had first appeared during puberty. There was also evidence that she had a special place in her handsome father's affections and that her mother played a subsidiary role in the family. There was a strong family history of mood disorders and alcoholism, stretching back at least two generations. When I tried to explore the meaning and impact of these revelations, Jane showed no interest at all in addressing the issues. More importantly, I was unable to convince her to begin eating a caloric diet. In desperation, I called a meeting of Jane's college roommates and enlisted their cooperation in monitoring her diet and urging her to gain weight. After a while they withdrew from the field of battle, overwhelmed by their sense of failure.

Jane, contemptuous of my ineffectiveness, walked into my office one day and presented me with a book by Steven Levenkron on treating anorexic adolescents.[6] She imperiously ordered me to "read it and do what the man says!" My interpretation of the author's viewpoint was that anorexics, far from rebelling against over-controlling mothers, had in fact been permissively indulged so that consistent limits had not been internalized. In consequence, their individual will had become grandiosely and destructively inflated. They needed to be disciplined and corralled, as if one were taming a wild horse.[7] I followed the new paradigm assiduously: I took Jane out of her group because of noncompliance with treatment recommendations, became more stringent about collecting professional fees, and insisted that she sign a waiver relieving me of responsibility in case of an adverse outcome. Soon thereafter, she started eating normally again. Her menstrual periods returned, and she began dating. After graduation from college, she became the manager of a highly regarded restaurant near campus. When last heard from, she was pursuing a career in restaurant management. Although happy about the outcome, I was mystified by how the steps I had taken led to the positive changes in Jane's behavior.

These two case histories illustrate a number of points. One of them, charitably put, is that I am not a conventional therapist. I am directive, prescriptive, and stage manager—all thought to be disqualifying activities for a reputable therapist. I bring in families and roommates to assist in the process, and I am not above trying to outmaneuver the destructive forces that cause symptoms, not just by relying on psychological insight but also by taking certain forms of forceful action. Although I value insight, I think other potentially more powerful therapeutic forces must be summoned. Of these, perhaps the most important is the patient's own will to health. In the first case, the will to health was so strong that once I broke through her hysterical coma, she performed a form of psychodynamic therapy on herself with no obvious prompting from me. In the second case, the patient actually provided me with a guidebook for her successful treatment.

Why do I say such behavior is a manifestation of a strong "will to health"? Why not attribute it to a strong drive or high motivation to succeed in therapy? Why invoke a quasi-mystical force such as "will to health" when more naturalistic, scientific-sounding terms such as "drive" and "motivation" would do? The answer to these questions gets at the heart of the main thesis of this book: that there is a need for a spiritual conception of therapy because the highest forms of physical and mental health can be truly understood and achieved only through adding the spiritual dimension to the usual medical and psychological approaches. By invoking the notion of a will to health, I am introducing a spiritual concept, a purposeful ideal, the first of many that I propose to use in going beyond biological, psychological, and social factors to get at the true complexity and richness of the forces manifested in falling ill and becoming well, in failing to develop maturity and then succeeding at it.

To clarify my purpose here, I want to describe a situation in which the absence or opposite of a will to health—the will to death—was manifest. Gary was a middle-aged man who was diagnosed with diabetes, adult type 2, and prescribed oral hypoglycemic agents. Although the likely long-term effects of uncontrolled diabetes were described to him, he disliked taking anti-diabetes pills and therefore stopped them early in treatment. A few years later he was on kidney dialysis for diabetic kidney disease and was practically blind from diabetic degeneration of the retina. When asked why he had stopped the medication, he replied, "I gambled, and I lost."

Instances of such self-destructive behavior are common in any medical or psychotherapy practice. We see patients who marry known thieves and then are devastated when their money is stolen, or patients who continue ice-climbing after already having suffered many falls and broken bones, or patients who won't stop smoking despite the proven risk of lung cancer. The subsequent funerals, attended by grief-stricken family and friends, are heartbreaking affairs. Less clear-cut is the case of an acquaintance who sought my advice about continuing his medication after recovering from a major depression. I strongly urged him to do so because, as I explained, relapses might start insidiously and be accompanied by accidents or self-destructive behavior rather than overt return of depressed mood. Influenced by another professional's strong bias against psychoactive medications, he stopped his Prozac and was killed in a bicycle accident a few weeks later. Sadly, these kinds of sequences—ending an effective treatment followed by a tenuously connected disaster—are not uncommon in clinical practice.

These are examples of what I consider to be the absence of a will to health, or what the Italian psychoanalyst Edoardo Weiss called *destrudo*, a death instinct. Since the notion of a destructive instinct or will to death hardly fits into the framework of science—it clearly belongs to the dark side of the spiritual realm—psychiatrists and psychotherapists who value their scientific credentials and reputation do not openly subscribe to this fanciful notion. They tend to have a mind-set that excludes such ideas from serious consideration. I want to trace the origins and underpinnings of the scientific mind-set before elaborating on the properties of the spiritual mind-set. But first, some unfinished business.

Meaningful Coincidences

I hope that it has not entirely escaped the reader's attention that there are some puzzling coincidences flavoring the clinical vignettes I have recounted. The hospital commander assigned me to the position of base psychiatrist without knowing that, after a bad turn at surgery, I was half-consciously wishing to return to my first love and my main reason for going to medical school in the first place: to become a psychiatrist. This fateful assignment fell right into my lap. It was so right that it proved to be a life-changing event.

Then my first patient as base psychiatrist recapitulated the general outline of my own prior therapy, betraying a knowledge of the process of psychodynamic exploration with neither the past experience nor the education to account for it. No doubt, she was naturally gifted and intuitive. But still, where did her therapeutic expertise come from? As demonstrated by my response, I had no idea and was obviously annoyed by her abrupt declaration of a successful termination. And then another patient, Jane, in whose treatment I was failing miserably, presented me with the guide to therapeutic success. How often does that happen in therapeutic relationships? Perhaps more often than we recognize.

Synchronicity and Serendipity

There are two concepts in general use that help to make some sense of such seemingly unlikely events: serendipity and synchronicity. Serendipity, a notion derived from a Persian fairy tale,[8] concerns the accidental discovery of something of immense value. Fleming's discovery of penicillin by noticing the effects of a contaminating mold on a tissue culture of staphylococci is a classic example of serendipity. Such discoveries are examples not only of valuable coincidences but also of an individual's capitalizing on such seemingly chance occurrences through a readiness to make the best of them.

In the examples cited previously, my assignment as base psychiatrist and Jane's gift of a treatment guide are good examples of occurrences that afforded me the chance to use them serendipitously.

Synchronicity is a broader concept of valuable chance occurrences. It is Jung's term for meaningful coincidences[9]—that is, concurrent events whose simultaneity is thought to be improbable or incomprehensible on the basis of scientific causality yet seem to be connected by meaningful purpose, or what Jung called an "acausal connecting principle." This purpose usually involves a great benefit to the one who experiences the coincidence, such as happened to me and my patients in the examples cited previously. Over time, I have had many more such experiences that I have sometimes been able to take advantage of. During the course of my own psychoanalytic therapy, I would often leave my therapist's office after an emotionally intense session to find my own next patient bringing up the same issues that I had been discussing with my therapist, whose responses served as good models for my own. Or I would suggest a somewhat obscure book for a patient to read only to have her produce it from her purse. Not to recognize, at the very least, that we were on the same wavelength surely would qualify as scientific fundamentalism, better known as scientism. By the same token, we should not overlook the possibility that the attribution of meaning to coincidences can be projected wishes that introduce personal bias into the field of observation. Serving heavy soups of such mercurial ingredients without adding large dollops of skepticism is a quick way to join the society of mad hatters. I am counting on my readers, as well as myself, to resist getting carried away by the phenomena alluded to in what follows. A strong will to believe often induces us to cherry-pick the data, ultimately leaving us with none of the weapons of rational analysis that are necessary to maintaining sanity in facing the dangers of the spiritual quest.

Other common synchronistic events are the following kinds of experiences: having memories or concerns about long-lost friends only to have them suddenly materialize or thinking about telephoning someone who has long been out of touch only to have him unexpectedly ring us up. Of course coincidences may be negatively meaningful as well, as in the mode of bad karma or "what goes around comes around." Sometimes schadenfreude, or delighting in the misfortune of another, even a supposed friend, is rewarded by a similar misfortune befalling oneself. If, as a consequence of such an experience, one becomes more empathetic toward others, then the meaning of the coincidence is transformed to a learning opportunity.

The coincidences of serendipity and synchronicity have no special meaning within the current scientific framework. They are mere curiosities. Faced with such occurrences, the contemporary scientist either espouses agnosticism about their purported significance or demonstrates by mathematical and empirical methods that their occurrence by chance is far more likely than has been assumed. At the opposite end of the spectrum, some religious people, especially followers of Alcoholics Anonymous, believe that happy coincidences are instances of "God acting anonymously."

My own position is that meaningful coincidences, since they involve teleological purposes, do not fit within the causal framework of modern science. To be sure, incidence and prevalence studies of improbable coincidences are legitimate subjects of science, as the work of Paul Kammerer[10] suggests, but their purported causes either are undiscovered or lie outside the boundaries of scientific reasoning. But they fit comfortably within the spiritual framework. In fact their occurrence is assumed to be one of the prime manifestations of spiritual influences at work. As we shall see, the bedrock of spiritual belief is that all minds, all instances of consciousness, are somehow connected to form one overall consciousness, which I call Spirit. And the empirical world is a projection or emanation of Spirit in its willful, creative mode. From this perspective, there should be little wonder that the aggregate of thoughts create events that mirror them and that what goes around from one mind comes around in other minds. The unity of consciousness entails that what happens to one of us happens to all of us, even if, in order to maintain sanity, we typically screen out any awareness of this interconnected reality.

As I will argue in later chapters, I believe that this screening process is a form of dissociation, whose very purpose is to avoid psychosis. Some instances of psychosis, characterized by a belief in thought transference, may be the unfortunate consequence of too much psychic porousness: the inability to filter out the psychic overload of experiencing all-consciousness. Jill Bolte Taylor's description of her success in mastering this experience as a result of a left-brain stroke, as described in her inspiring memoir, *My Stroke of Insight*, is a daunting example of the possibility of gaining prime spiritual awareness.

> My left hemisphere had been trained to perceive myself as a solid, separate from others. Now, released from that restrictive circuitry, my right hemisphere relished in its attachment to the eternal flow. I was no longer isolated and alone. My soul was as big as the universe and frolicked with glee in a boundless sea.[11]

The problem with having this openness to spiritual truth is implicit in the discussion: without great care and training—a process Plato called habituation, related to what I later (chapter 9) term creative dissociation—it can easily lead to psychic disintegration and the inability to function in the everyday world. Plato alluded to this possibility in his *Allegory of the Cave*, which describes our everyday experience as no more than the shadow projections on a cave wall of a higher light, the true reality.[12] Being forced to look directly at the light of reality without habituation would be so painfully blinding that we would no longer be able to see and function in the everyday world. So it is understandable that we flee desperately back to the shadowy projections of the empirical mind-set. Not only is it productive of the empirical associations and judgments that allow us to survive and prosper in the sensible world, but it can be a bulwark against creeping psychosis. With these ideas in mind, I want to draw out the distinction between scientific and spiritual reality by describing the origins and tenets of the empirical mind-set.

Scientific Empiricism

Most educated people, in leading their everyday lives, take for granted a belief in scientific empiricism. This roughly says that facts and theories have to be supported by repeatable empirical observations and controlled for subjective distortion to be considered objectively true. In the absence of such confirming observations, assumptions about reality have no objective status.

Right at the beginning of modern science, William of Occam (c. 1288-c. 1348), a late medieval monastic philosopher, advised us to invoke the fewest possible causes to explain reality. This so-called principle of parsimony further maintained that only *individual* things or beings exist; supra-individual forms or universals have no extra-mental existence. In keeping faith with such notions, modern scientists are the intellectual offspring of this Benedictine monk. As opposed to postulating a Platonic heaven from which ideals of beauty and truth somehow shape our abstractions from experience, present-day empiricists say the process goes the other way around: we derive these abstract notions of beauty and truth simply by repeated experiences of beautiful things and truthful statements and noting what they have in common. There is no need to postulate an influential realm that lies outside experience. Just stick to the facts of experience, ma'am!

In establishing their empirical credentials, these hardheaded, sometimes cold-hearted, left-brained linear thinkers claim to be "shaving Plato's beard with Occam's razor." They ask, "Why postulate the existence of entities that lie outside the realm of ordinary sense perception, like Plato's ideals and so-called spiritual truths, when you can explain, predict, and control your interactions with the everyday world without recourse to them?" The only acceptable answer is that the entities *exist* and can be directly experienced by the prepared right-brained, parallel-processing mind even though the evidence for them may not meet the standards of scientific truth. And for those who have the means of repeatedly experiencing them, there is no doubt that they exist, anymore than there is doubt about the value of great works of art. Great plays are not just collections of great lines, and great music is not just a linear collection of great tunes. They also have ingenious structures that embody and communicate experiences of great meaning and truth. No matter that empiricists who do not share this belief claim that such experiences are illusions or even hallucinations, not justified by the sense-data. The spiritual therapist maintains that those who have these experiences in forms that do not compromise their ability to function in the everyday world are provided with a richer, more fulfilling, and healthier life than those who do not. It is a supreme irony that Occam declared that religious and spiritual truths, though not provable by human reason, were given by Revelation! If by Revelation, he meant spiritual awareness, in principle available to us all, then we should not blame *him* for the cherry-picking of his beliefs by modern scientists.

Spiritual Knowledge

The truths of spiritual knowledge go beyond the testimony of our senses and conceptual organization. For a person to arrive at spiritual truth, empirical knowledge must be complemented by the givens of intuitive awareness. Since these intuitions are notoriously vulnerable to subjective distortion, they must be subjected to critical analysis. This includes ferreting out the personal needs that might distort spiritual intuitions and anticipating the behavioral consequences of acting on them. Only then can they become reliable guides to living right.

Scrubbed of distortions, intuitive knowledge yields the answers to the fundamental spiritual questions of what is the ultimate truth, what is our fate, and how should we live. All the right answers are connected to the central intuition that we each have a higher self or soul that links us all together, the aggregate of which constitutes the ultimate reality: the universal will, or Spirit, and its ideals. Whether this is premise or conclusion, getting at the component answers and acting according to them is what leading a spiritual life means. What kinds of answers have passed the test of time, and what kinds have proved to be fool's gold?

The spiritually aware are not disposed to accept simplistic slogans that reduce everything to the biology of instinctual behavior or the psychology of pleasure-seeking and pain-avoidance. We look beyond simple explanations in search of deeper, often hidden influences and meanings. In the spiritual aspect of our lives, we resist the temptation to shave Plato's beard with Occam's razor. We believe that the bushier the beard—and the more moss on the rolling stone—the richer the life. So we shy away from formulations such as the following:

1. Altruism is just a manifestation of having "selfish genes" or a survival-of-the-species instinct.
2. Moral behavior is nothing more than learned behavior or a manifestation of what our "gut instincts" tell us or, as in number 1, what is most geared to individual and group survival—to inclusive fitness.
3. Religious faith is an immature, neurotic set of beliefs attesting to a thumb-sucking need for comfort in the face of a dangerous existence.
4. A belief in rebirth or an afterlife is nothing more than a denial of the inevitability of death.

Even though there is a measure of truth in each of these assertions, none of them speaks the whole truth. Filling out the picture requires the addition of spiritual brushstrokes.

In making the transition to positive beliefs, we must note that adopting the spiritual viewpoint and leading a spiritual life does not commit us to believing in the God of formal religion. To the seeker of spiritual truth in my sense, the existence of an all-powerful, all-knowing divinity stretches beyond the intuitions of spiritual awareness. Instead, we affirm the existence of Spirit or Soul, a nonpersonal organizing force that we can connect to and be influenced by, without believing that it intervenes in our lives. In truth, becoming spiritual may necessitate a rejection of the formalisms of past religious training, although we may retain a measure of "religious" faith by transforming some of its tenets. Whether or not we believe in the existence of the biblical deity, following the spiritual path does require a belief in something beyond ourselves and our egocentric interests and intelligence. What this something more is has been described in many different terms, including God terms.

The French philosopher Henri Bergson (1860-1941) said it was the *élan vital*, or life force, that was pushing toward a purposeful creative evolution, not just a blind biological one.[13] In a similar spirit, Pierre Teilhard de Chardin, a French priest and paleontologist, thought this evolutionary force, which was essentially evolving from mind to spirit, was undergoing a cultural convergence toward a conscious global unification of human awareness.[14] However one conceives of this spiritual force, the aim of spiritual therapy, as here conceived, is for both patients and therapists alike to attune themselves and contribute to the progressive flow of Spirit. In the chapters that follow, I will try to explain what this means and draw out the consequences for a comprehensive therapy of human beings, who are nothing less than spiritual beings.

Consequences of Spiritual Knowledge for Therapy

The main consequence of spiritual knowledge is that therapy becomes a spiritual undertaking: a process of coming to exemplify the highest moral-spiritual values. In this process, the therapist must prove worthy of serving as spiritual guide or mentor, whose example and advice the patient freely seeks and freely chooses to follow or not to follow, without fear of rejection. Far from being a blank screen or a morally neutral analyst of projected wishes, the spiritual therapist must be able to offer not only technical expertise, which may in fact require a temporary or occasional stance of moral neutrality, but also and more importantly the knowledge and life experience that lead to the wise value judgments for which there is no ample empirical evidence. In other words, the spiritual therapist must have the wisdom to know that we can never derive what ought to be from what is. The leap can be made only by good judgment that takes account of individual needs and values, social context, empirical knowledge, and universal ideals.

Chapter 2
THE SPIRITUAL FRAMEWORK

Summary. After providing a clinical illustration, I define some of the key attributes that spiritual therapists must be able to identify and promote. These include the will to health, the true self and its guiding spirit, character, empathy, intuition, artistic expression, finding a calling, and ultimately connecting to the one, all-embracing creative consciousness: intelligent, willful Spirit. This connection infuses us with spiritual values and confers a sense of blessedness: the gratitude of being alive in a meaningful universe. I then explain how the spiritual framework provides the ultimate goals and values for the medical and psychosocial approaches to therapy and inevitably introduces value judgments and prescriptions into every aspect of diagnosis and treatment. For example, value assumptions determine whether we diagnose someone as depressed or rationally bereaved and therefore the type of treatment, or no treatment, we recommend. Evaluation and objective choice are fundamental to the scientific-empirical approach to therapy, and inspiration and guidance are the additional ingredients of spiritual therapy. Choice of treatment has much to do with the patents' (and therapists') tolerance for suffering and the effects of its presence or absence on their creativity and spirituality. Scientism and psychologism are anti-spiritual over-elaborations of the scientific and psycho-behavioral frameworks, respectively. The domains of the medical and psychological clinical sciences have to be delimited to make their goals amenable to spiritual guidance. Once this is done, the way is open to healing body, mind and spirit.

The Case of Carl

I first saw Carl for long-standing symptoms of depression when he was in his mid-twenties. He lacked spontaneity, had few interests, and spoke in a hollow voice. He went through the motions of trying to sell real estate. He had only a few close friends. Moreover, he felt alienated from his small family: a mother, sister, and two cousins. In Carl's early adolescence, his father committed suicide. His sense of loss was compounded by the guilt of having angrily yelled at his father a few days before the tragic event. Afterward, he no longer enjoyed his former pursuits. He had been a good athlete, especially at playing baseball; now he could no longer "hit the ball," his description of his general loss of competence and vitality.

In the following months Carl was told by family acquaintances that his father had been involved in a fraudulent insurance scheme, and at the time of his death he was being threatened by both law enforcement and his criminal associates. Magnifying Carl's loss, his guilty, humiliated mother transferred him out of his middle school and the family's synagogue, which separated him from his two main social networks. The change of synagogues was especially painful because he had been devoted to his religious studies and teachers. Then his mother married a European businessman, who moved the whole family to Germany, where Carl did not speak the language and was hurt by the perceived antipathy of classmates and neighbors.

Back in this country, his college experience left no strong impression except for a single event: driving back to school from visiting his first and only college girlfriend, he fell asleep at the wheel and woke up on the side of the ride, thrown clear of his totally wrecked car. Miraculously, he escaped with only minor injuries. Accidents proved to be part of a pattern: his every attempt to have a relationship with a woman had a self-destructive outcome. Returning from a date in New Jersey, he fell asleep driving across the Benjamin Franklin Bridge and smashed into the guardrail. Another time he fell off his bike, suffering many cuts and narrowly avoiding a collision with a passing car. Often he would have to terminate dates because of nausea and abdominal cramps.

Fearing for his life, I intervened decisively in several ways, starting with suggesting he hold off on further dating and giving him phone access to me whenever he felt in danger—temporary measures until we could neutralize the mortal danger he apparently faced. At the same time I expressed hope and caring by praising him for his resilience and courage in surviving his traumatic past and by reassuring him that he would get better because he was a survivor, that he seemed to have a guiding spirit that protected him from serious, irreparable harm. But we couldn't afford to continue tempting the fates. I also made it clear that we would have to work hard to understand the sources of his self-destructive behavior and to develop strategies for overcoming them. He committed himself to the program.

Appreciating that he needed to be in a more energetic, hopeful psychobiological state to endure the approaching ordeal, I started him on an antidepressant regime of medication—which quickly improved sleep, libido, and confidence—and cognitive-behavioral therapy,[15] involving regular exercise, the elimination of negative thinking, and an active search for more meaningful work. Concurrently we explored the psychodynamics of his irrational belief that he caused his father's death at a time of his burgeoning adolescent sexuality and the resulting guilt that interfered with his expression of normal masculine aggression, sexual vigor, and a sense of competence and worth. We also affirmed that he harbored an "internal saboteur" because of a dissociative split in his personality (discussed further in later chapters). We explored how this dissociation had been traumatically induced in adolescence and served the purpose of warding off a psychotic reaction to his traumatic losses. We also discussed a strategy for corralling his saboteur and getting it to work *for* him instead of against him.

Finally, I prescribed two courses of action. First, despite his initial resistance, I persuaded Carl to join one of my groups. The purpose was to overcome his isolation and to garner the necessary support for restoring his damaged morale, which involved coming to believe in his worth and ultimate success in earning a life worth living. He also needed the shared wisdom and caring of colleagues who could show him the principles and means they had found useful in overcoming self-destructive behavior and finding the path to a fulfilling life. My hope was that his tapping into the group spirit would persuade him to break out of old patterns and take the risks of developing new, more productive ones. While in the group, Carl fell in love with a fellow group member. Everyone pulled for the success of their relationship; it was the group's baby. They were disappointed when I invoked group rules against romantic and business relationships among members and therefore insisted that at least one of them leave the group and either stop group therapy entirely or enter one of my other groups. They chose to be in separate groups to take advantage of the continuing support and guidance the group work offered.

Group support and monitoring combined with specific treatment approaches enabled them without further incident to get married and to have three children. In the search for a meaningful career, Carl decided to emulate a respected family friend by getting a degree in social work and taking a job in a hospital. He soon discovered that he was unsuited for clinical work. Every time one of his patients showed significant signs of depression and hopelessness, he would panic and become paralyzed with fear of an impending suicide. We ultimately decided that it was not worth the time and effort to overcome this residual post-traumatic symptom since in even "safe" cases, he experienced little joy in the work. However, in the course of trying clinical work, he became interested in the business side of providing social workers to local health care facilities. To prepare himself for developing such a business, he earned an MBA through night and weekend classes. He subsequently built a successful social work agency in the Philadelphia area. To ensure high performance levels among his professional workers, he instituted teaching programs targeted to promoting spiritually healing values and the specific skills they would need for their various assignments. Making a success of this social work and home health care agency became an all-consuming, gratifying process, well suited to his interests and values. He started innovative social work clinics in rural areas and organized team home visits to de-escalate dangerous family situations, both audio-visually supervised from distant locations by clinical experts.

My second suggestion to Carl was that despite now being a professed atheist, he should join a synagogue. My aim was not that he would come to believe in the existence of a personal God, much less that he should become an observant Jew. Rather, I wanted him to repair the hole in his being that had resulted from his early losses—most importantly, his father and his ethnic-religious affiliation—and that had destroyed his sense of having a whole, true self. He had become a hollow, deracinated person, a state of non-being that in my opinion no amount of medicine and conventional therapy could ever repair. To be sure, some of the infusion of Spirit that he needed might come from working with a caring therapist and spiritual group. But considering the earlier painful loss of religious affiliation, he also needed to reconnect to the rich ethnic heritage that a welcoming synagogue might provide.

I referred him to a congregation that was known to embody strong social values, to practice *tikkun olam*—Hebrew for "repairing the world"—and to have a highly spiritual rabbi. I daresay that the events that followed could not have been readily predicted by anyone, certainly not by me; I was operating on a hunch and a hope.

When Carl introduced himself after the first Sabbath service, the rabbi seemed to sense the nature of his distress, for he quickly walked him to his office where they could speak in private. The rabbi was moved to tell Carl that he too had lost his father to suicide. He spoke of seeing his father on his deathbed and watching life flow out of him, leaving behind an inanimate body. Because of this experience, he had come to believe in the existence of a spiritual reality that was the animating force of earthly life. He also had come to realize that his father was ill and that he, the rabbi, bore no significant responsibility for his suicide, and he was certain that the same was true for Carl. In saying so, the rabbi enhanced the process of relieving Carl of his burden of guilt and unworthiness, an unburdening that Carl connected to his subsequent development of a sense of goodness and purpose and a less diminished ability to love and receive love.

This conclusion was foreshadowed by what happened on the way home from this deeply meaningful encounter with the rabbi. In a state of heightened awareness, Carl by chance spotted a row house on fire. Seeing fire and smoke emanating from a second-floor window, he jumped out of his car to assess the situation and then called the fire department. While awaiting the firefighters' arrival, he alerted all the people in the house and guided everyone to safety except those trapped on the third floor. The firefighters arrived in record time and were able to rescue the rest of the inhabitants, among whom were small children. Carl departed the scene with a great sense of satisfaction and the blessed feeling that the gods were in his corner, an "illusion" that I was happy to reinforce.

The next phase of his treatment involved gaining greater control over his residual internal saboteur. During times of stress, this split-off subpersonality continued to punish Carl rather than aggressively confront others who might be mistreating him. Foremost among his tormentors was his wife, who began to blame him for all problems in the family. Under this daily barrage he developed severe symptoms of depression. Unable to follow the suggestion of his group to get out of the line of fire by moving into a hotel, he continued to passively absorb abuse. I made it clear that I could no longer take responsibility for his welfare if he did not take action. Under this pressure, he agreed to a conference including his wife and her current therapist (she had fired me earlier when I would not approve her going off medications). The family meeting dispelled his fear that his wife would commit suicide or suffer a breakdown if they separated. Although the subsequent divorce was less than amicable, Carl came away feeling whole and justified. He said he was able to "hit the ball" again. He found a more suitable, loving mate and expanded his health care network to provide the kind of innovative services for poorly served populations that gave him the sense of practicing *tikkun olam*.

Artistic Ramifications

One of the most interesting aspects of Carl's integration of his true self and his finding a calling was a spontaneous manifestation of artistic talent. One day he showed me beautiful sketches of his children and public figures. Having had no idea that he possessed such skill, I was stunned by the accuracy and expressiveness of the drawings. I encouraged him to pursue this avocation by taking studio classes and seeing what he could learn from studying the past masters of painting and drawing. He was not interested. He had no intention of learning the techniques to become an accomplished artist. Rather, he used his artistic activity as a way to playfully express his raw creativity and his newfound interest in the character displayed in the faces of others. He ultimately devoted a good portion of his downtime to portrait-sketching, with increasing satisfaction and refinement in the work. This became his meditation, yoga, and prayer: it allowed him to achieve a heightened sense of focused awareness, and the focused attention was effective in relieving him of the accumulated stresses of a very complex love and work life.

In the process of undergoing spiritual therapy, many patients, especially those with a past history of artistic or musical accomplishment, return to these forms of expression with enhanced interest and satisfaction. My office walls are filled with drawings and paintings they have made. Many of their group colleagues are also recipients of this creative largesse. These reawakened artists typically attest to the benefits of their artistic activities in terms of enhanced, focused awareness and diminished anxiety and depression.

The Practice of Spiritual Guidance

From the perspective of conventional practice, this once again is a highly unorthodox form of psychiatric and psychotherapeutic treatment. It explicitly acts on moral-spiritual values to treat a patient in a caring way and to prescribe courses of action leading to a good life: to be true to oneself, to develop the strength of character to say both yes and no in the service of gaining authenticity and wholeness, and to find the kind of work and love relationships that yield a calling and a sense of blessedness. More specifically, I would make the following points.

To do effective spiritual therapy, therapists must use their own spiritual sensitivity to promote the spiritual growth and health of their patients. As we saw in chapter 1, this involves recognizing and maximizing their will to health. In Carl's case, this was a dire necessity because he harbored a self-destructive partial self that at times threatened to overpower the self-protective will to health of his true self. The latter needed to be buttressed and amplified by a therapist-ally who appreciated both aspects of Carl's character: both his will to health and his death wish. Therapists who are insensitive to the workings of these conflicting spiritual agencies are prone to dispensing their treatments, whether biological or psychological, in an objective manner that fails to communicate that they are joining their patients in the life-versus-death fight for their bodies and souls.

Patients in whom the will to health is weak tend to show resistance to following treatment plans, even manifesting conscious self-destructiveness, as in continuing to smoke, overeat, use narcotics, and drink and drive recklessly despite obvious potentially dire consequences. They do not take their medications, or they fail to perform mutually agreed-upon assignments. In such cases therapists must do nothing less than, by whatever means short of physical coercion, persuade them of the necessity of compliance if they are to succeed in turning their lives around. Doing so requires not only giving care and hope but also describing in vivid, arresting terms the consequences of making or failing to make life changes. By calling a fear-reducing marital conference and questioning the usefulness of continued therapy unless he took action, I set limits on Carl's self-destructive behavior and enabled him to terminate a failed marriage. This pitted two competing moral values against one another: honoring marital vows versus ensuring psychological and spiritual survival. The patient concurred in judging the latter to take priority in this case, even after taking account of the harm that a broken home would inevitably inflict on his children.

The "will to health" is only one of many spiritual terms that come into play in this type of morally infused therapy. Following are some of the others:

a. The *true self,* equivalent to the higher self, typically lies deep within the individual's unconscious mind, often in embryonic form; it has the potential to connect with all manifestations of consciousness and ultimately to Spirit or the life force. Intuitively gifted individuals may be prompted by the conscience of their true selves at an early age, sometimes without the usual suffering and hard work that are the typical entrance fees.

b. The *guiding spirit* is the active agency, the will, of the true self that protects individuals and keeps them on the path to finding and developing their calling, often yielding uncanny synchronistic events that serve as potent reinforcers.

c. *Character strength* concerns the person's steadfastness in manifesting identity, loyalty, and high ideals—a set of attributes that may not be realizable without repairing dissociative splits in the self and engaging in gymnastics of the will.

d. *Empathy* enables a person to intuit and appreciate the feelings and values of others and to see the world from their perspective. From a universal perspective, compassionate empathy transforms others into parts of oneself and oneself as a part of others.

e. *Intuition* is the gift of knowing, beyond an exclusive reliance on sense perception, what people are feeling, thinking, and planning and what has happened or is about to happen in the world. Caring about these individuals and the fate of the world yields compassionate empathy.

f. *Finding a calling* transforms a job or the exercise of a profession into the expression of one's strongest interests and talents in the service of contributing to the repair and betterment of the world.

The Purpose Amplified

From the spiritual perspective, the overarching purpose of life is for each of us to realize our potential by connecting to the true, higher self—the portal to Spirit itself—and in the process realize to the fullest the other spiritual attributes that flow from it. Manifesting these qualities is tantamount to repairing and developing the self until it merges with Spirit, in the process contributing to making the empirical world a morally purer emanation of Spirit. To the extent we succeed in this task, we achieve something greater than happiness. We come to feel blessed to be alive, for we have become aligned and even merged with the flow of Spirit, which is equivalent to partaking of the wisdom and energy of higher awareness, of becoming part of the universal will. This is blessedness in its fullest meaning, for it allows those who share in it to understand and even welcome with joy both the euphoria and the suffering of the biological cycles of living and dying.

Spiritual Therapy as Integrative and Corrective Treatment

Before we discuss the practical application of these notions, I want to place spiritual therapy in the context of other standard forms of mental health treatment. In making the case for a spiritual therapy, I am obviously not arguing against other standard approaches, which I respect and use where appropriate, as I did in Carl's case. Rather, I am making the case for integrating them within a larger moral-spiritual framework. My main reservation about these other approaches, particularly the pure medical and psychological models, is that they sometimes pretend to an objectivity and comprehensiveness they do not possess. Their practitioners make assumptions that, once examined, reveal their biases and limitations.

For example, diagnosing depression and prescribing antidepressant medications are assumed to be straightforward, value-neutral scientific operations. But this position can be sustained only through failure to examine what assumptions have been made about the valid criteria for diagnosis and treatment. For example, even in the last thirty years, the criteria for diagnosing and medicating depression have drastically changed. What used to be considered normal variations in mood and temperament, such as shyness, pessimism, grief reactions, and winter "blues," have now become clinically diagnosable disorders, a fact that has drawn harsh criticism from some theorists.[16] What many of us have difficulty recognizing is that our standards of health have evolved. By raising the bar for normality, we have lowered it for abnormality. Whether we judge this to be a good thing or a bad thing (I think it is on balance a positive development when properly applied, as I think it was in Carl's case) is largely a question of values, particularly the moral-spiritual values that address the question of how we ought to lead our lives.

Our current diagnostic expansionism and therapeutic activism clearly imply that the best life is the one with the fewest symptoms and restraints on self-achievement. The less the amount of suffering, the better the quality of life. But in its raw form, this is surely a position open to question. And in fact it has been questioned in vigorous terms.[17] Reasonable people holding different values strongly disagree about the answer. Although it would seem that terrible, prolonged mental and physical pain ought to be avoided when possible, how are we to reconcile this position with the contributions of great leaders and artists such as Gandhi, Lincoln, and Beethoven, whose suffering was of no lesser magnitude than their achievements? Is it likely that they would have made the contributions they did if they had been relieved of their symptoms at the start? Or were the symptoms and contributions inseparably linked?

To be sure, this kind of thinking is hard to accept when we are faced with the unbearable, intractable physical and mental pain that we ordinary mortals not uncommonly suffer. But should we not take such questions into consideration in deciding about the treatment of lesser degrees of pain that have the potential to induce greater awareness and creativity? I believe we have to calculate the benefits versus the risks, the upside versus the downside, every time we propose to relieve artists of mood swings at the expense of their art or to relieve the faithful of the dark nights of the soul that inform their faith. We therapists have seen moody writers lose interest in writing once lithium tamped down their mood swings. The tides of inspiration no longer come in or go out.

Only rarely in standard discussions of psychiatry and psychotherapy are these issues confronted head-on. Many of us are only dimly aware of how much we take for granted in giving or accepting not only a diagnosis but also a recommended treatment. We gain greater awareness when we consider the following questions: To alleviate psychiatric symptoms, is it really better to take medication than to engage in vigorous exercise, hard work, psychological uncovering, or meditation and prayer? Or is it better to do some or all of them together? Instead of recognizing that these are questions to some extent about situational values and therefore can never be answered definitively, we give ourselves the illusion of objective knowledge by making prior assumptions about empirical legitimacy, in the process narrowing the boundaries of acceptable "facts."

Unacceptable Notions

If we speak of a prophetic dream or of a "guiding spirit" in the person of an Air Force colonel directing us to our calling as psychiatrist or in the person of a rabbi who helps replace a self-concept of a destroyer with that of a savior—as happened to me and Carl, respectively—we are regarded either as unhinged or, if among friends, as having overactive imaginations with a penchant for science fiction. Heaven forbid that we should profess a belief in the reality of the paranormal or the supernatural. Those who consistently beat the bank at gambling casinos are just called lucky. But the managers of these casinos know better. The culprits are either expert card counters or just plain "hot." The managers don't wait until the luck of these consistent winners might revert to the statistical norm; rather, they usher them off the premises as soon as possible.

And think of leaders with great charisma who have led masses of people to great feats of creation, like Washington in the founding of our nation (Joseph Ellis in *The Founding Fathers* describes scenes in which bullets seemed to be repelled by the exposed general leading his colonial troops forward), and others who have commanded such widespread allegiance that followers have carried out orders to commit genocide or cultural annihilation, such as Hitler in the devastation of Europe and Stalin in the extermination of the Polish and Ukrainian intelligentsia. I think that all three of these leaders possessed "paranormal" powers, one for good and two for evil. What is the ability to hypnotize a crowd, even a whole society, to do one's extraordinary—sometimes good, sometimes evil—bidding if not paranormal? It hardly needs saying that such an idea is not susceptible to scientific validation and has no place in objective, empirical discourse.

But in limiting the realm of legitimate observations, we also make unprovable assumptions about what experiences and procedures are acceptable. This is obviously the case when we reject claims of uncanny coincidences or presumed clairvoyance. But we overlook the possibility that differing values and assumptions may be at play in less egregious disagreements about the facts. For example, studies purporting to show the superiority of a medical technique over a nonmedical one or vice versa in treating, say, depression, commonly make different assumptions and follow slightly different procedures, sometimes out of unrecognized bias, but often out of different notions about diagnosis, adequate treatment (cognitive therapists have often used suboptimal types and doses of antidepressants in "proving" the superiority of their approach), and criteria for improvement—phenomena derived more from different values influencing what is actually observed or, more fundamentally, what is in principle observable or unobservable.

In stressing these points, I do not wish to deny that at some point in time a consensus about optimal treatment, such as a combination of drugs and a specific nonmedical psychotherapy, may be reached. But just as certainly, at another time new recommendations will be made, perhaps because of a paradigm shift,[18] based not just on new discoveries and observations but also on the fact that different perspectives embodying different value assumptions have been adopted. And these new assumptions inevitably shape the observations in new ways. Think about how our notions of a well-played basketball game have changed as players have become faster and shown greater athleticism and especially since the introduction of the three-point shot in the NBA in 1979. Successful teams have come around to playing a more wide-open brand of basketball, recognizing that making one-third of three-point shots (the league average is actually above 35 percent) is as good as making one-half of two-point shots, which is a higher rate than most teams achieve. As a consequence, the average number of three-point shots taken in the NBA has quadrupled in the past two decades. No team can consistently win without a number of good long-range shooters. Lovers of basketball tradition say that the game has been ruined, that new players know only "run and gun," not the sound fundamentals of the game.

These kinds of considerations clearly apply to classical psychodynamic assessments and treatments. We do not accept the validity (note the value word) of their claims without sharing their assumptions about the characteristics of maturity and normal sexuality, and also about the status of religious faith. Classical psychoanalysts have tended to ascribe healthy normality to heterosexuality and atheism and pathology to homosexuality and religious faith. But these are quite clearly assumed values belonging to past times rather than well-supported facts about optimally productive behavior, as suggested by the now-greater acceptance of homosexuality and same-sex marriage as normal variations rather than pathological conditions. If we substitute spiritual awareness for religious faith, I am convinced that therapists of the present who may be generally sympathetic to psychoanalytic thinking, as I am, are much less likely to label believers in a spiritual reality as developmentally arrested than was the case even in the recent past. Different values, different realities.

I think our reluctance to examine such value assumptions derives in part from our habitual resistance to changing old ways of thinking. But it also comes from fear of the consequences of admitting that most of our important decisions are based at least as much on value judgments—on "good judgment"—as on solid empirical knowledge. In the heat of having to make the myriad choices and to take the multiple actions that daily living requires, already difficult enough, we would be paralyzed if we had to remind ourselves that at every turn we are flying by the seat of our pants, relying heavily on our fallible judgments in the absence of clearly posted directions. Imagine sending a lapsed Catholic back to church or a lapsed Jew back to synagogue on purely scientific grounds. On what basis? Mainly, because in the case of

Carl it seemed the right thing to do, not because a few poorly designed studies suggest that the faithfully observant are happier than their opposites.

In the pages that follow, I do not try to hide from these recognitions. Instead I embrace the position that the most meaningful aspects of therapy lie outside science to inhabit an artistic-spiritual realm. I maintain that scientific knowledge, certainly important and basic, is just the foundation on which successful therapy rests. Vastly more important to achieving the highest form of mental health is the superstructure: spiritual knowledge and practices that lead to stronger and truer character, empathy, core values, and callings. These are all spiritual attributes whose development is necessary to achieving integrity of the soul. Let us remind ourselves once again that the original meaning of psychotherapy is the healing of the soul. In making my case, I rely heavily on our best intuitions and judgments about who we really are and what we ought to do. As I have made clear, I do not think these intuitions are entirely reliable. Ultimately their truth must be subjected to critical thinking, checked out by experience and buttressed by as much empirical knowledge as we can muster.

The Quest for a Theory

We currently lack a comprehensive theory of psychotherapeutic change. The medical, psychodynamic, cognitive-behavioral and social models all make significant contributions, but each model gives only a limited view of the extraordinary complexity and multiple determinants of human behavior. By placing the moral-spiritual dimension as the keystone of the whole arch of human development, I hope to make some progress toward formulating a theory that does for the twenty-first century what psychoanalytic theory did for the twentieth century—that is, to provide a guiding framework for our understanding of how our past endowments and experiences have led to our current predicaments and how they can all be transcended to redeem the true self and its connection to Spirit. First, we must examine an important distinction.

Evaluation versus Inspiration

The possibility of doing spiritual therapy requires us to make a distinction between two radically different approaches to promoting greater mental and physical health. I contrast them as the "mode of evaluation" versus the "mode of inspiration."

In the mode of evaluation we use the scientific method to measure objectively to what extent the psychiatric therapies are beneficial. We adopt a skeptical attitude toward claims of efficacy. We use blind experimental controls to screen out the influence of subjective expectations on the comparative outcomes. When the treatment agent, such as a new antidepressant medicine, significantly exceeds the benefits derived from a placebo, then we conclude that the antidepressant is biologically effective. This result is never easy to come by because the placebo effect can sometimes account for 30 percent or more of symptom betterment. Often, to demonstrate a "real" effect beyond the placebo, the number of experimental subjects and controls may have to be laboriously large. Sometimes a new medicine must show significant benefits in more than 60 percent of subjects for the evaluators to accept it as truly effective. Ideally, these evaluators should have no personal stake in the outcome, but in an imperfect world, we accept the next best case: that the experimental controls are tight enough to prevent the evaluators' biases from grossly influencing the results, or so we presume.

In taking the second perspective, the mode of inspiration, we enter an entirely different world. Here we are in the realm of the therapist as healer rather than objective scientist. True healers, though they rely on the results of scientific studies in selecting and prescribing a treatment, offer treatment not with a skeptical or wait-and-see attitude but with the full force of their persuasive personalities.[19] They want patients to get better with all their might. They lend their own faith in the treatment to enhance the basic pharmacological, psychological, or behavioral training effects. They willfully contaminate the objective efficacy of the treatment by moral suasion—that is, by the inspirational force of their own faith in it. Another way of looking at this approach is that the healer uses the placebo effect to positive advantage rather than regarding it as an unwanted contaminant. Of course, to retain credibility, the healer might in passing admit that the treatment does not work every time, only enough of the time to inspire hope and faith.

In the inspirational mode of the healer, we recognize that faith and its positive expectations play a crucial role in treating body and mind. Yet despite a mountain of evidence in support of this claim, we rational beings of the twenty-first century are loath to admit its truth because it leaves the door open to quackery, to unwarranted claims for all kinds of worthless elixirs and purgings.[20] Those of us who have had home remedies applied to infections and lacerations by well-meaning mothers and grandmothers, our own home-based faith healers, know of the dangers firsthand. So let us quickly slam the door on the potions of snake-oil merchants who make unwarranted claims on their behalf. To retain our intellectual integrity, we must insist that although faith can be an enhancer of objective effects, we should never rely on it to the exclusion of the search for scientific validation.

Yet in a technological age that has spawned remarkable new treatments for some of our most debilitating maladies, we are tempted to overvalue biological discoveries and to minimize the effects of faith or its absence. We may do this despite having repeatedly witnessed how pessimism, negative expectations, or nihilistic lack of faith—augmenting the so-called *nocebo* effect—can defeat even the most objectively potent treatments, just as positive expectations can maximize the weakest ones.

For example, Mr. Alexander, who worked on the power lines in my hometown, was grazed by a downed hot wire, and barely escaping death by electrocution, he suffered a disfiguring, painful injury to his right hand and arm. Now partially disabled, he could no longer perform the job that gave him a sense of worth. As a result, he stopped being the friendly, cheerful man the townspeople had always known. But then to our surprise, he abruptly became his old friendly self again, albeit now a bit unsteady of gait and speech, once he began taking the patent medicine Hadacol. As most adults growing up in the teetotalist South in the middle of the last century would know, Hadacol was an alcohol-laced (24 proof) liquid of no known therapeutic value beyond the effects of its base spirits. It was promoted as a panacea for many poorly defined psychosomatic conditions, such as "lumbago" and "rheumatism." Calling Hadacol a placebo, a neutral-sounding term used primarily in scientific studies, does not do justice to the contagion of faith that it inspired, its "curative" powers dramatically promoted by the touring "Hadacol Caravans" that came through practically every town in the Deep South. Having long ago given up on the healing powers of his religion, Mr. Alexander was now a devout worshipper at the altar of the Hadacol services, which were nothing less than pseudo-medical revival meetings. Would he have done better if there had been a Prozac Caravan in his time? Instead of a nonspecific patent medicine, a biologically effective antidepressant promoted with religious fervor—doesn't this strike a contemporary chord?—might well have given benefits without the loopiness induced by Hadacol.

The inescapable conclusion is this: in matters of health and disease, strong expectations of a positive response to treatment are crucial to getting the best possible results. A good inspirational therapist wants to capitalize on good science and good faith at the same time. However it is achieved, a 30 percent or greater boost in efficacy is not to be lightly dismissed.

Parameters of Faith

What kind of faith are we talking about? The word "faith" usually evokes the notion of belief in a supreme being who has the power to right wrongs, heal the sick and maimed, and sustain a personal relationship with the faithful. And to be sure, religious faith of this kind may help people shoulder the inevitable burdens of pain and loss in the temporal order. But the intellectual spirit of modern times derides this brand of faith. At the heights of religious fervor in the past, many placed their hopes for salvation in a divine order that would see them through the dark passages of suffering. Although this fortress of faith may have been partially breached by the encroaching rationality of the Renaissance and the Enlightenment, it was not generally questioned by the majority of the populace until the first half of the twentieth century. The destruction of the great wars, culminating in the firebombing of Dresden and the atomization of Hiroshima, along with the genocides of Armenians, Romas, Jews, and other ethnic groups—still going on to this day in parts of Africa, the Middle East, and Asia—shook the bastions of religious faith, at least in the Western world, to their foundations. Given that these cataclysms were soon to be accompanied by advances in scientific understanding and information technology making it possible to have an hour-by-hour and minute-by-minute account of practically all the natural and human disasters afflicting the whole earth, it has become difficult for even minimally skeptical people to retain substantive faith in the existence of an omniscient and omnipotent being who answers prayers and caters to the sick in body and soul. After Nietzsche's declaration that "God is dead,"[21] what powers or principles are we to believe in to provide a structure of meaning for our catastrophe-ridden lives? Fortunately and unfortunately, as we shall see, other edifices of faith have been erected to supplement or, in many cases, entirely supplant the tenets of formal religion.

Chesterton said that people who don't believe in God are liable to believe in *anything*. He perhaps forgot to mention that people who *do believe* in God are also liable to believe in anything, whether or not connected to their religious faith. Granting Chesterton the possibility that the need for religious-like faith is inborn and therefore subject to dangerous miscarriages when it is denied, we note that some atheistic men and women of the twentieth century were forever evangelizing for nonreligious faiths that were no more rational—and in some cases vastly more destructive—than the depredations of fundamentalist religion. In the case of the state totalitarianisms of the Nazis and the Communists, not even the Inquisition and Crusades came close to matching them in sheer human and cultural annihilation.

But what about the other replacement faiths, perhaps more benign and therefore liable to have a more insidiously widespread effect? Among all the pseudo-scientific belief systems that have sprouted up over the years, I single out not just the political fundamentalisms of the radical left and the radical right (Tolstoy condemned them both, saying the difference between them was merely the difference between dog shit and cat shit) but also the one-issue fanaticisms such as found in some right-to-life adherents who are opposed to contraception even to prevent the spread of sexually transmitted diseases and pregnancy termination to save the mother's life. And what about the consequences of faith in far more subtle belief systems, such as scientism and psychologism, which call for critical dissection because they have made unjustified and harmful claims to comprehensiveness?

Scientism and the Repudiation of Spiritual Truth

Scientism, an outgrowth of too many close shaves with Occam's razor, is an excessive faith in the process and fruits of scientific discovery. It maintains that the only truths worth knowing are the products of scientific investigation. In one of its most sophisticated formulations, logical positivism,[22] it proclaims that the only meaningful statements are those that are empirically verifiable, or in a later refinement, empirically falsifiable.

Just a moment's reflection reveals the reductionist absurdity of this position. There are truths of the heart and truths embodied in myths, legends, poems, and spiritual testaments that are meaningful but in principle not verifiable or falsifiable. They contain the intuitions and moral and aesthetic judgments, assuredly not divorced from empirical antecedents and consequences but not accounted for by them alone, that guide the major decisions of our lives, such as whom to marry, how to raise children, whom to trust, and finally, what to believe in. Better and worse judgments are fundamental to such decision making, even though there will always be room for disagreement about what we did or did not do or should do in the future.

The guiding themes of the Hebrew and Christian Bibles and their commentaries provide the literary foundations of the moral code and practical standards of behavior for the whole of Western society. In particular, the Talmud, comprised of rabbinical interpretations of the Hebrew Bible, and subsequent writings of medieval seers like Maimonides and the author(s) of the *Zohar*, offer practical guidance on all aspects of daily life.[23] They tell us what values to inculcate in children (respect for elders, gratitude for life's benefits, generosity even to strangers), how to conduct business fairly, and what beneficent care we owe to the natural environment and its inhabitants. These are answers to the pragmatic question of how to live the right way that confronts us at every turn of our march through time. Granted that some of the venerable prescriptions may have been superseded by the phenomena of biophysical and cultural evolution, for us to conclude that the spiritual truths of earlier times are not worth knowing about, as believers in scientism are likely to attest, is the height of narrow-mindedness. Undoubtedly, such impoverishment of thought was at work when the faculty committee charged with changing the core curriculum at Harvard College recently voted against including a course on "faith and reason" as a basic requirement, instead substituting an exploration of "what it means to be a human being"! (See *Harvard Crimson*, December 13, 2006.)

Is the study of the history and tenets of religious faith, the inspiration for much of our finest art, architecture, literature, and music and the Western moral code, unworthy to stand alongside the history of science as a basic requirement of a Harvard-educated person? Scientism, here a narrow, exclusionary belief system about what knowledge is "real," seeks to marginalize the fruits of humankind's long, glorious struggle to make sense of the cosmos and the challenges of everyday living, the distilled wisdom that addresses the real requirements of being a good and healthy human being. The written word and the oral traditions of our Western religious heritage, sometimes taken literally, sometimes metaphorically, contain legends and commandments that have guided generations of human beings along the path of a spiritually balanced life. The hunger for this kind of wisdom, to correct our tendency to be nonjudgmental about pervasively lax standards of child-rearing and family life—no structure; no accountability; no shared meals, activities, or decision making—goes a long way to explaining the widespread popularity of a book such as Wendy Mogel's *The Blessings of a Skinned Knee* (see footnote 23 above), value-permeated advice to the modern family based on Talmudic wisdom. Having lapsed in observing many of the crucial values of our own spiritual traditions, we try to impose these very same values on alien cultures without any longer living them ourselves. The hypocrisy is glaring, as is the inevitable failure of such projects.

Making good choices in the absence of all the facts separates the wise from the foolish. Some of us clearly show better judgment than others, and each of us does better at some times than at others. Although very few therapists, not to mention hard scientists, would be willing to admit it, almost all these judgments concerning our most important life decisions derive more from our values and intuitions than from our empirical data and therefore have a large moral-spiritual component. When we try to figure out which path to take, we are basically trying to determine the right thing or the best thing to do. And we often have to ask ourselves, "Best for whom?" When does the common good trump the rights of the individual, and vice versa?

To be sure, the answers cannot always be stated in absolute terms; often they must be taken as provisional hypotheses. Yet we are certain that Lincoln made the right choices in abolishing slavery and preserving the Union, that Gandhi obeyed the highest moral principles by starving and martyring himself to establish Indian independence, that Sakharov and Solzhenitsyn showed great courage in accepting the consequences of exposing the cruel despotism and thereby hastening the demise of the Soviet Union, and that Mandela earned the praise of all humanity by averting a blood bath in South Africa, even after his cruel, long imprisonment would have demanded retribution from a lesser person. And we have no doubts that Hitler, a dark embodiment of evil, did virtually nothing right except build good roads. These conclusions we take on faith, on trust in the validity of our moral judgments. We presume them to be self-evident.

What I want to show in this book is that the main choices we have to make in doing psychotherapy, whether as patients or as therapists, have no less a moral-spiritual, value-judgment dimension than our other important life decisions. Only rarely is our field of action delimited enough for scientific knowledge to prove decisive. We are almost always falling back on faith in our intuitions and value judgments. Not only is that the way it is, but that's the way it has to be, once we grant the incompletability of our knowledge and the existence of free will, which carries with it the obligation not to escape from freedom,[24] but to do everything we can to free our will and use it wisely.

If there were a self-revealing deity, we would have no reasonable choice but to have religious faith. Similarly, if we always waited to have definitive scientific knowledge about consequences before making decisions, we as rational beings would certainly choose to follow the course that the empirical facts and laws dictate, especially if the benefits and costs were agreed upon. But the matter is almost never so simple; the costs and benefits are themselves often points of contention, as in the debates about the facts and causes of global climate change. Out of necessity we are forced to become moral as well as scientific empirical agents. Otherwise, we might already have agreed to slap a large tax on gasoline consumption, to provide incentives for building and taking rapid public transportation, and to build more renewable fuel power plants than are currently operational. Adopting these policies will never be determined by scientific findings alone. But as of now, I am convinced they are the right ways to go and worth fighting for.

Such policy proposals expose sharp disagreements about their inherent values, about the acceptable risks and benefits they would variously entail. Even though we are now getting closer to acknowledging that global warming is real and that the human contribution is significant, the proposed remedies continue to foment a gridlocked moral and political debate with no end in sight. This is likely to remain the case unless and until a series of worldwide climatic catastrophes, already underway, forces us to come to our senses and take action. As I write this in the aftermaths of hurricanes Katrina and Sandy and the typhoon in the Philippines, we are hopefully getting closer to "facing facts," which means recognizing that the facts are subject to value assumptions and commitments.

Psychologism

The free will issue, as formulated in the theory of psychic determinism, exposes a major deficiency of psychologism, especially in its orthodox Freudian formulation. As someone who reveres Freud's genius and values my personal psychoanalysis, I feel no conflict in decrying psychologism as a system of thought while still appreciating many of the achievements of the psychodynamic approach. "Psychologism" refers to an extension of Freud's insights about psychological development and unconscious motivation that lays claim to a comprehensive theory of the etiology and treatment of human neurosis. A popular form of this theory claims that neurotic symptoms are caused by early, mostly repressed experiences and conflicts (psychic determinism); that symptomatic cure is most effectively achieved by gaining cognitive-affective insight into the causative effects of these early experiences (cure through psychological insight); and finally, that spiritual and religious beliefs are infantile, neurotic symptoms, compensatory in nature, that function as resistances to true intellectual-emotional insight (religious and spiritual beliefs as symptoms of arrested psychosexual development).

Not only has this approach turned out to be of questionable value in practice; it also has had deleterious cultural consequences. Genetic and pharmacological discoveries have repeatedly demonstrated that although psychological factors are rarely unimportant in the genesis of human neurosis, they are often secondary to genetic-biochemical factors. And although psychodynamic insight is often helpful in giving focus to therapy, it is only rarely definitive in overcoming symptoms, whereas medication often combined with cognitive-behavioral learning and psychological insight often are. And by making the moral-spiritual life wholly a function of childhood psychic determinism, and a neurotic function at that, true-believing practitioners of psychologism have deemphasized the character, intuition, and empathy of patients as the moral bases of choice, once neurotic symptoms are overcome.

Yet because the psychologistic way of thinking was the dominant influence on most forms of therapy and psychosocial philosophy for most of the twentieth century and continues to be, if now to a lesser degree, it has had a major retardant effect on the incorporation of both biological and moral-spiritual factors into therapy. Up until very recently, most therapists felt a sense of failure if they had to medicate a patient. It meant the patient or therapist wasn't up to finding the true psychological causes of symptoms, and the patient was therefore being consigned to a lesser form of treatment. A few boats carrying Thorazine and Tofranil over from Europe in the late 1950s, some lawsuits over the withholding of medication in suicidal and homicidal patients, and restrictions on insurance reimbursements for multiple therapy sessions per week, all radically altered this way of operating, if not the thinking behind it.

But more importantly, because psychologism has typically been anti-spiritual and therefore provided little basis for moral behavior beyond early conditioning and rational analysis—even the possibility of an inborn conscience has been considered more of a liability than a gift—it has had an even more disastrous impact on the spiritual life of psychotherapy patients and the culture at large. How do you get from *what we do* to *what we ought to do* on purely psychological terms? The psychological answer would have to be something like enlightened self-interest or "stop ruminating!" Thousands of years of moral inquiry—all the way back to Moses, Socrates, and Jesus and up to Maimonides, Kant, Rawls, and Parfit—thrown onto the soft low couch of pre-genital sexuality! But really, once we stop being neurotic, how should we live? Is it all a matter of gaining instinctual gratification and staying out of trouble? As the once popular song asked, "Is that all there is?" Do we find ourselves washed up on an alien shore, not knowing why or how we got here, with no goals other than survival and socio-economic advancement? Settling for such a nihilistic philosophy of life is surely taking the path not to realism but to cynicism and despair.

Spiritual Guidance

In the spiritual therapy that I propose, psychiatrists and psychotherapists earn their professional fees not only by technical competence but also by expertise in moral and spiritual guidance. No nondirective nonsense except as a temporary strategy for promoting self-reliance, out of the humility of genuine ignorance, or as an acknowledgment of our patients' inborn and hard-earned rights to self-determination. The therapist worth more than a beginner's fee has expertise to share, an expertise born of broad experience in living and making practical and moral choices. In this book, I propose to ground a theory of prescriptive psychiatric treatment in spiritual values that must be infused by the caring guidance of real people in real relationships. My view is that psychotherapy must be true to its word: it must be a therapy of the soul, a spiritual treatment that leads to a meaningful life. I want to show that each person has a true self, a core being that may have been compromised by biological errors and early conditioning but that can be discovered and brought forth by repeated acts of will, once the biological and early learning deficits are repaired. In the process the person's character is fired and formed in the crucible of painful, transformative experience. This means that the individual develops the wherewithal to stand firm and remain faithful to the core values of the true self, despite private recriminations and even public opprobrium. Armed with strong character, individuals and groups can then become more meaningfully spiritual by progressively attaining empathetic, constructive attunement, first with family and love partners and then progressively with friends, strangers, and the living world, all of whom become subjects of caring reverence.

What this formulation means and how it is carried out are our main concerns here. By concentrating on the core spiritual values of character, empathy, and finding and developing the true self and its calling, I aim to place other effective psychiatric treatments in context. The pharmacotherapies and the psychotherapies—in individual, family, and group formats and in psychodynamic and cognitive-behavioral modes—are conceived as some of the means to achieving a true and meaningful life permeated with spiritual values. In the process, the formation and development of a spiritual group are shown to embody the essence of this approach and one of its most far-reaching fulfillments.

Spiritual therapy draws inspiration from Maimonides's account of character but goes on to amend it by saying that we form our character and choose our own way by repeated acts of will, *once our will has been freed up to act*. This is what a spiritual therapy, at its best, offers those who are suitable for it and willing to do the arduous work it requires.

The Better Times

If there is no good time to suffer from mental or physical illness, I believe this is an especially hopeful time in human history. The discoveries in molecular biology, neuroscience, public health, infectious disease, immunology and chemotherapy of malignancies, medical and surgical treatment of cardiac and circulatory pathologies, and the biology and pharmacotherapy of mental illness have all contributed to a climate of optimism that we will conquer the great physical and mental scourges of human and animal life. These discoveries have also given us a better idea of where science leaves off and spiritual commitment must take over. The good psychiatrist and psychotherapist can now offer a medically and psychologically informed approach to treating mental symptoms and, at the same time, recognize that human beings do not live by empirical truth alone but must tend to the higher realm of spiritual truth. I propose a spiritual therapy that is pro-science but seeks to go beyond science without losing respect for all forms of knowledge and for traditional moral and spiritual values as well.

Chapter 3
PERSONAL DIMENSIONS OF SPIRITUAL THERAPY

Summary. I describe an adolescent reaction to racial prejudice that facilitated my recognition of a spiritual realm of values that greatly influenced my later work as a physician and psychiatrist. I saw that patients had not only chemical imbalances, psychological conflicts, and faulty learning; their suffering also carried a deeper spiritual meaning that had to be understood and developed. Yet such conscious experiences are not a prerequisite to becoming a spiritual therapist. In fact, many therapists do spiritual therapy without recognizing it as such. Even the most basic function of the psychiatrist, performing the psychiatric evaluation, is often done in the spiritual mode by humane therapists. By way of a case example, I delineate the differences between symptom relief, psychological growth, and growth in moral and spiritual awareness. Spirituality in modern terms is distinguished from traditional religious belief and from ordinary psychological awareness. I acknowledge Freud's role in cleansing spirituality of its irrational contaminants—a tribute that he might regard as meager indeed. Aside from such age-old practices as meditation and prayer that induce spiritual awareness, there are also spontaneous spiritual experiences, such as one's reaction to artistic and moral profundity, that open the doors to higher consciousness. The conundrum of identity and its relationship to choice of profession, sexual orientation, and the formation of a false self are also subjects of discussion.

An Experience of Racism and its Consequences

When I was twelve, I found myself seriously at odds with my family, classmates, and teachers about how black people were treated in our small town in the Deep South. I felt ashamed when they were called "dirty Ns" and thrown into jail for drunkenness by the town marshal, who doused them with whisky to prove his point. I could not understand why most of my family did

35

not share my sense of injustice. Were we not also members of a persecuted minority whose people were still being exterminated in Europe? Why did the townspeople not see that these black people were poor and in need of help? Not exactly appreciated for my moral insight, I was excited to go off to a New England boarding school at age fourteen. My parents were greatly relieved to get me out of town before I did serious damage to their social and business interests. What seemed remarkable to me and my new classmates was that I, hardly a model of courage and no stranger to racist feelings in myself, was seized by a sense of moral outrage that virtually no one around me shared. Before national legislation and media coverage of the integration movement, I had no access to the growing national sentiment except perhaps to the occasional article in the magazines to which my parents subscribed.

How did I come by my conviction of racial injustice? I hardly measured up to the character of truly courageous white Southerners. In the 1930s, Arthur F. Raper, a sociologist from North Carolina, was forced to leave his academic post in Georgia for taking his students to visit a black college; in his writings he depicted the tragedy of lynchings in the South and shone a light on the exploitative nature of sharecropping. Juliette Morgan, an aristocrat from Montgomery, Alabama whose parents were friends of Scott and Zelda Fitzgerald, was so horrified by the mistreatment of Southern blacks that she mounted a lifelong crusade against racial injustice, supporting Rosa Parks in her stand against segregated busing and serving as one of the inspirations for Martin Luther King's crusade before she was driven to suicide by the white backlash against her passionate advocacy. In the aftermath of World War II, William Hodding Carter II, editor and publisher of Greenville, Mississippi's *Delta Democrat-Times*, fought for the rights of Japanese-American citizens and denounced a local chapter of the White Citizens Council for its persecution of African-Americans, enduring public vilification and death threats as a consequence.

Beyond foolishness, why would someone like me take such a vocal anti-racist stand, without the courage and strength to stay and fight for it. Of course there were predisposing psychological determinants: oedipal, pre-genital, and no doubt factors farther back and forward beyond. For any number of reasons, I strongly identified with the black help who were often overworked and underpaid. As I later understood, empathy for others, a key spiritual attribute, played a part in my animosity towards racial persecution. But in truth, just like my family and townspeople, I also harbored prejudices against black people. I differed from many of them in feeling that it was wrong to have such feelings and even worse to act on them. Something kept me from always yielding to my worst instincts, rather than listening to the conscience of my higher self. I could not keep quiet about the mistreatment of these people whose main "black mark" was their dark skin color. Somehow I knew they deserved to be regarded as fellow human beings. I knew this because something inside told me so, no matter what anyone else said, just as I later came to know that certain pieces of music (Bach, Mozart, Beethoven) and literature (Sophocles, Tolstoy, Dostoyevsky) were profoundly great, no matter what others, among whom were esteemed critics, might think.

Personal and social outrage over instances of racial prejudice and mistreatment of the poor and the weak that cannot be entirely accounted for by past learning has led others like me to believe in the existence of a spiritual conscience that transcends the effects of genetics, psychological conflicts, and social conditioning. To be sure, the strength and influence of this transcendent moral conscience vary greatly, evident in some as a weak infrastructure requiring repeated and costly learning experiences to develop into a reliable structural determinant of behavior. But in the spiritually gifted it makes itself known early in life as a solid foundation that requires few environmental stimuli to be developed in the character structure of individuals and, by extension, in the values of groups of which they serve as influential members.

Fortunately, Thomas Jefferson and our other founding fathers manifested this heightened conscience in the national sphere, if not always in their private lives. Even some of those who were slave owners recognized that all people are born equal with inalienable rights to life, liberty, and the pursuit of happiness. And these ideals *are* self-evident truths to those with a strong moral sense. Much to be admired are their later advocates like Abraham Lincoln and Lyndon Johnson who displayed the character strength to further the process of making them real in our nation as a whole.

Those endowed with a strong conscience—which is sometimes no less a curse than a blessing—are often moved to take a stand against prejudice and ethnic hatred. They know in their hearts that these injustices violate the fundamental principles of right and wrong and the sense of justice embodied in the Declaration of Independence, the Golden Rule, and "the categorical imperative."[25] Racial prejudice, the intolerance of differences among people, and the blaming of victims instead of taking responsibility for our own victimization of them are some of the common denominators of these wrongs. Persecution and mass murder springing from intolerant religious fundamentalism are salient examples in these times of religious terrorism and tribal genocides in many parts of the world.

But race and religion are not the only magnets attracting these malignantly destructive attitudes and their crusading proponents. Differences over politics, sexual orientation, marriage equality, abortion choice, abstract art, and even the value of psychiatry and psychotherapy continue to generate religious intensity, pitting seemingly rational people against each other in undying enmity. Recently, in a fit of righteous intolerance, a celebrity actor, a member of the Church of Scientology, publicly condemned a fellow actor and the psychiatric treatment she had undergone for postpartum depression. The intolerance behind such attempts at character assassination and debunking of medical science by people of influence must be curbed if progressive societies are to develop their full potential—or even to endure.

Spiritual awareness prompts us to stop harming, deceiving, and coercing others and to stop wantonly indulging appetites for materialistic pleasures at the expense of spiritual values even though most everyone around us is doing it and egging us on to follow suit. The implications for spiritual therapists are manifold. Not only must we exemplify these qualities in our therapeutic and other personal relationships, but we also must guide patients to adopt them and make them part of their character structure whenever feasible. Of course, good timing and sensitivity to capacities for change are essential to success. The necessary spade work has to be done before we push for abstinence from addictive, self-destructive dalliances and games. And we should save our strongest persuasive bids for the big stuff, such as striving to become loyal and faithful to loved ones and charitable toward those needing forgiveness and material and spiritual help. We push for these value changes because we know that we and our patients can never achieve psychological and spiritual health so long as we indulge in behavior that caters exclusively to our egocentric needs, for in doing so, we destroy our connection to Spirit and thereby lose our moral integrity.

Equally important, we must recognize and show appreciation when a patient spontaneously moves in a spiritual direction. A sudden awareness of having crossed the moral line prompted one of my formerly homeless patients to abruptly stop taking and dealing drugs and living off the handouts of churches. In the middle of hustling a church in the Midwest, she said, "I realized I had gone too far—it just wasn't right and could only lead to my total ruin." She left her group of stoned merry marauders and called her parents for a plane ticket home to New Jersey. A few years later, she had earned her

MSW and developed a successful practice treating wayward adolescents, about whom she knew more than could be learned from books and classes. I recognized the strong underlying character and moral conscience that enabled her to make unaided changes of this magnitude and worked with her both individually and in group to build on this foundation to become more caring and proficient in her work and in her personal relationships. I came to respect her moral guidance system enough to take seriously some of her many criticisms of me—she was a tough customer to put it mildly, early on accusing me of being "the good doctor who is trying to fuck with me"—and not to be content with always attributing them to transference reactions.

So as we set out to do spiritual therapy, we must develop not only techniques for behavioral change but also the empathic attunement that leads us to treat others compassionately and the sense of values that guides them (and us) to seek lives of meaning and moral integrity. In so doing, we gain greater understanding of our patients, and we earn the chance to provide spiritual role models for them to emulate. Moral intuition also helps us understand how those endowed with a strong moral sense, without adequate family and social support to develop its rudiments into workable programs for living, may become estranged from mainstream society and find their way to self-destructive and antisocial behavior patterns. For them moral treatment is not just the therapy of choice; combined with medical and psychological techniques, it may be the only effective treatment. Only spiritual therapists are able to provide the support and appreciation that the morally and psychologically gifted need to overcome the damage to their higher, spiritual self resulting from having been raised by people who failed to appreciate and nurture their unique qualities.

Fortunately, the moral-spiritual qualities required to do this kind of repair work do not have to be advocated or even consciously held to be manifested as a healing force by well-trained, naturally caring and empathetic therapists.

Spiritual Therapy as Humane Therapy

The happy truth is that good therapists do spiritually informed therapy without necessarily realizing it or labeling it as such. They are likely to profess their commitment to the standard psychological therapies, in either psychodynamic or broadly eclectic forms. But to the extent that they think of their work as embodying humane values, such as treating patients with caring concern, spiritual ideals are certain to enter into the work. I hope to demonstrate this point by describing how experienced, caring therapists typically approach their patients with an eye to honoring and elaborating the spiritual dimension.[26]

The Initial Clinical Interview

Humane therapists typically begin the work by assuaging patients' distress. We do this by establishing rapport and conveying hope. Rapport is achieved by manifesting an attitude of sympathetic understanding, typically without taking notes in the beginning or in any way diverting attention from our fellow sufferers as they sit in front of us and tell us why they are seeking help. Whenever possible, we let them know that we empathize with their suffering, that we don't blame them or think them weak for developing symptoms, and that even with modest prognostic signs, we have confidence they will get better if they work hard at making changes. We do what we can to change their attitude from pessimism to reasonable optimism. Above all, we show appreciation for who they are and what they are going through, not failing to note special character traits such as courage and perseverance, always present in those with a strong will to health and moral character. Conversely, we are attuned to signs of a broken will and the resulting weakness of character as variously manifested by failures of conviction and resolve, patterns of self-defeat, and drug- and risk-taking addictions.

Then we ask patients to tell us more about themselves: precisely what kinds of symptoms they have, when these started, what brought them on, and what made them better or worse, including past treatment. We ask about their families and whether any of their relatives have suffered from similar or other psychiatric conditions. We also want to know about the quality of their relationships with parents, siblings, and spouses and whether these types of relationships tend to be repeated in their romances, friendships, and work life. Did their major role models hold steady as objects of respect, or did they suffer debasement, either by their own or by society's wrongs—for example, by loss of position or status or even life itself? How did such outcomes affect patients' self-esteem and sense of belonging and feelings of blessedness?

We want to know if they have suffered early losses or traumas and if these have led to recurrent patterns of failure and loss. We also want to know if they have had any serious illnesses, accidents, or treatments, such as surgeries or chemotherapies, that have had long-term consequences. We also inquire about their philosophy of life and its underpinnings in religious and secular values. As spiritual therapists, we try to assess the adequacy of this philosophy as a guiding belief system and an effective curb against loss of morale or the lure of criminal, immoral, and self-defeating patterns of behavior. Finally, we examine their cognitive abilities and affective responses and determine whether specific inadequacies indicate that further studies are needed to rule out conditions that might hamper their chances for leading a worthwhile life. Somewhere along the way, we make a provisional diagnosis— that is, we determine whether the array of symptoms and findings cluster into recognizable syndromes such as disorders of mood and cognition, pointing the way to the best paths of treatment, to interventions that increase the chances of leading a life of optimal gratification and sense of accomplishment.

Since the formal wording of diagnoses, as found in the APA *Diagnostic and Statistical Manual*,[27] can be needlessly alarming to patients, we are apt to share with them a formulation in lay descriptive terms, such as "illogical thinking," "low self-esteem," "mood swings," and "harsh self-criticism," instead of such terms as "psychotic thought disorder" and "major depression" or "bipolar depression," unless they are already comfortable and personally familiar with these clinical conditions. When it seems appropriate, we also discuss the patterns of behavior that seem to get them into trouble and also the possible role of genetics and traumatic past experiences in causing or sustaining these patterns—all of which has the added advantage of absolving patients from excessive self-blame and sense of failure. Of utmost importance, we strive to state the particulars of the formulation in a way most likely to convey relief, hope, and support in a shared undertaking. By so doing, we have the best chance of securing their informed consent to follow an often arduous proposed treatment plan. Then, in formulating the treatment plan, we discuss in a preliminary way some of the difficult choices that may have to be made to achieve a good life: some of the activities and associations that may have to be changed and the moral resolve that may be required for them to do so effectively.

Note that the caring attention that goes into this kind of work is already a spiritual phenomenon. It wouldn't be quite the same if done by a detached evaluator anxious to avoid revealing anything about his own past struggles—even less so if done by an interactive computerized voice, the assuaging automatons of the banks and other institutions that field our telephone requests and complaints. If we manifest genuine, individualized caring empathy in our every interaction with patients right from the very first contact, then we have a chance not only to reduce symptoms and change self-defeating behavior patterns, but also to promote a life-enhancing embrace of spiritual ideals.

One consequence of taking a spiritual approach is that patients often are inspired to change their lives fundamentally and sometimes abruptly once they feel really understood and appreciated. Sometimes they can do this without recourse to more specific and lengthy therapeutic interventions. As I suggested in chapter 1, some patients with a strong will to health can seemingly diagnose and treat their conditions all by themselves. I later recognized that this impression did not take account of the curative effects of even an initial encounter with a therapist who listens carefully and with evident human compassion. Perhaps good therapists unknowingly convey this healing spirit to patients who seem to cure themselves with only minimal apparent therapeutic intervention. I believe this happens more often than we acknowledge or even suspect.

If symptoms are not sufficiently allayed by rapport and spiritual connection and the psychological understanding that comes from the historical review and formulation, then we consider the advisability of specialized techniques such as medication, focused insight therapy, cognitive-behavioral therapy, hypnosis, biofeedback, and whatever other methods have shown consistent success in changing feelings, attitudes and behavior.

Symptom Relief

If medication is appropriate and the patient is amenable to drug therapy, then broad-gauged therapists try to find medicines that allay suffering and shorten the recovery process. But this medical part of the work, despite exciting advances in the past half century, is only one among many approaches, each perhaps with different goals. Drug therapy is primarily targeted to symptom relief, to diminishing the discrete manifestations of anxiety, depression, mania, cognitive disorganization, and various abnormal attitudes and behavior patterns, such as obsessive-compulsive traits. Since all these symptoms contribute mightily to the sum total of human misery, I do not wish to diminish the importance of any technique—medication, insight and interpersonal therapy, cognitive-behavioral learning, meditation, prayer—that might allay the suffering associated with symptoms and loss of morale.

At the same time we must ensure that recommending medications or other interventions is not done in an overbearing way that threatens patients' sense of autonomy, especially when their will might have been previously damaged by coercive parenting in early life or socially sanctioned violations of personal liberty and well-being. Sensitivity to such individual needs may necessitate taking medications off the table entirely or delaying their prescription to a later time in therapy, when character and will have been strengthened to the point that informed consent can be truly given.

Psychological Growth

In my opinion, good therapists, whether medically trained or reliant on medical colleagues, regard psychoactive medications and other techniques of symptom relief as adjunctive treatment, as a means to the end of a higher goal of treatment, usually termed psychological growth. This is growth and development in a range of personality attributes, the most important of which are these three: the capacity to take active and effective initiative; the achievement of the kind of self-control and self-reliance that confer independence and reliability; and the forging of non-self-centered relationships that temper egocentricity and allow the development of healthy interests in other people, activities, and social causes. Success in this venture is usually discussed in terms of the person's growth in the achievement of intimate relationships, career satisfaction, sustaining interests, and good citizenship. Although not always easy to achieve, the values inherent in these goals are easily understood, as the following vignette illustrates.

Max, a highly successful, compulsively busy real estate agent, was so involved with the academic and athletic success of his teenage son that he complained to the soccer coach about his limited playing time and stood over him every night as he did his homework, instilling in his son fear that he would not otherwise get into a top-rated college. Although a very bright, sensitive man, Max's reading was confined to business topics, and his recreation mostly involved occasional vacations at expensive resorts, which left him feeling gouged and empty. Max's diagnostic evaluation revealed a lifelong syndrome of anxiety and low-grade depression, punctuated by panic attacks, ruminative fears of bankruptcy, and bouts of harsh self-criticism. Both his father and his mother were plagued by anxiety and depression, suggesting a possible genetic component to his symptoms. Feeling less symptomatic on an antidepressant and focused insight therapy, he chose to work on psychological growth, defined as becoming less consumed by work, learning to treat his son and wife as separate people rather than as extensions of himself, and widening his interests to include diversified reading and enjoyment of films, music, and theater. None of this came easily to him, but he made the effort and began to enjoy a richer life. He equalized his relationship with his wife, and they began to share in making the important decisions of their family life.

In this case, we encounter a successful man who was nevertheless symptomatic and arrested in his psychological development. Once his presenting symptoms of anxiety, obsessive rumination, and depression were allayed, he elected to work on his psychological growth, which involved individuating from his wife and son and widening his interests. He set aside time in his schedule to pursue his new interests and to develop more mature relationships.

Spiritual Growth

But symptom relief and psychological growth do not exhaust the possibilities of therapy. With my support, Max also became interested in the values inherent in his work and his attitude toward the purpose and meaning of his life. By his own account, he was too competitive to enjoy anything but winning and too aggravated by the unethical behavior of his competitors to completely relish his successes. He wanted to change his outlook so that performing an honest service for his clients while being appropriately compensated became his all-important goal. In the process of realizing this ideal, his life became more meaningful. He eventually became delighted by his son's pursuit of his own interests and values (rather than following a track Max had imposed), which he accepted as worthy of respect. And he derived great satisfaction in helping clients find the right property at the right price, which often involved steering them away from less appropriate investments that might earn him a larger fee but would likely prove to be of lesser value to all concerned in the long run. He saw that any short-term financial sacrifice would be more than compensated by the goodwill of satisfied customers, who would more likely refer their colleagues and friends to him. You might say this is only good common-sense therapy or good business ethics. I would agree. It *is* good common sense and good business ethics, morally and spiritually good.

Therapy as Value Change

Although it is underappreciated, good therapy seeks to promote value change in patients. The assumption behind this goal is that much of human misery derives from having a belief system that is inadequate for coping with the losses and gains, the ups and downs, of everyday life. The good therapist tries to promote this change by helping patients address the issues of what must be done to find joy and peace of mind and what realistically to expect from people, including oneself, and from life in general. By themselves, accruing wealth, winning competitions, and seeing one's children get into the best schools and make the most enviable marriages will not lead to contentment. In fact irreversible despair might be the perverse outcome of meeting these goals.

It is by no means rare for individuals to commit suicide shortly after realizing their purportedly fondest dreams. They get their doctorates, generate fabulous wealth, make great discoveries, become leaders of institutions, and then promptly shoot themselves in the head or jump from the roofs of buildings. As is well known, this very course of events ended the life of one of the great leaders of American psychiatry just as he ascended to the summit of his profession.[28] Sometimes the great stress attendant upon great success precipitates a major depression or other malignant syndromes, physical and mental, that lead to these appalling outcomes. Whether or not we take clinical disorder as a given in such cases (I usually do), I think there is more to it. And in my experience this something more is spiritual emptiness: a lack of spiritual resources or, in what amounts to the same thing, the failure to develop the sense of self-worth that comes from a connection to a higher meaning of life. What a terrible personal crisis to achieve the outward accoutrements of worldly success and still feel worthless, hollow, and meaningless! Averting such an outcome is the proper domain of spiritual therapy. Symptom relief, psychological growth, and spiritual connection—these are the elements of a comprehensive, inclusive spiritual therapy that insures against bankruptcy of the soul.

Spiritual Crisis

Coming clean about the important role of spiritual values in effective therapy is especially important at this time because we have just come through one of the most harrowing spiritual crises in human history. The twentieth century was notable for its loss of spiritual moorings. I am speaking of a widespread loss of faith in enduring values, culminating not only in rampant materialism and exploitation of the weak and needy, but also in the kind of tribal and religious fanaticism that has resulted in repeated genocides and the destruction of whole cultures. In our horrified reaction to these cataclysms, we seem to be moving into a new spiritual age—at least, I hope this is so—in which it is no longer acceptable to avoid coming to grips with spiritual values in human and societal change. We are beginning to recognize that human beings are fundamentally moral and spiritual beings, and their spiritual aspirations must be realized for the highest forms of mental and physical health to be reached—for individuals and society as a whole.

Spirituality in Modern Terms

When spirituality is discussed nowadays, psychologically-minded moderns do not usually do so in conventionally religious terms, which may have unwanted connotations of dogmatic rules and rote rituals. Rather, we are more likely referring to qualities that we find in those we esteem most highly: the moral and aesthetic values that they manifest and to which we aspire. In becoming more spiritual, we are trying to live "the right way," to treat others fairly and in general to lead a good life. We want to feel that our existence has special meaning, that it serves a worthwhile purpose, that it is no chance occurrence that ceases to matter when we die. We want to value each human life—in fact, all living things—as uniquely varied manifestations of the life force or the one consciousness in which we all aim to participate. The belief that we are all united to form one Self is the very essence of what it means to be spiritual and is the source of our highest value: that we must do right by others; we must treat them as we would have them treat us because, like brothers and sisters, we are all the emanations of one whole Self with the potential to become fully conscious and active on its behalf. In doing so, we work on realizing our highest ideal: to become more "godly." Thinking in such terms makes us grapple with the necessity of recognizing a power or principle more important than our individual needs and plans. Those with religious faith call this higher consciousness God. But in this nonreligious discourse, I want to speak of this transcendent agency as Spirit, the unified higher Self or Will. Whatever we choose to call this higher consciousness or life force and wherever we "locate" it, either inside or outside ourselves, or *nowhere* in space and time, the recognition of its existence and its power to influence our lives makes us spiritual aspirants. Great scientists recognize this power no less than great artists and humanists. This is how Einstein put it:

> Everyone who is seriously involved in the pursuit of science becomes convinced that a spirit is manifest in the laws of the Universe—a spirit vastly superior to that of man, and one in the face of which we with our modest powers must feel humble. In this way the pursuit of science leads to a religious feeling of a special sort, which is indeed quite different from the religiosity of someone more naïve.[29]

Einstein said that this recognition comes with the feeling of the mysterious, which is "the fundamental emotion that stands at the cradle of all true art and science." His contemporary Ludwig Wittgenstein said we cannot speak meaningfully and clearly about such matters and therefore should remain silent. In writing this book I have voted with heart and soul for Einstein, whose intuitive gifts made him one of the greatest intellectual pioneers of human history.

The Hallmarks of the Spiritual Life

But what are the specific hallmarks of a life of spiritual meaning? First of all, those who serve as our best exemplars manifest core values that are relatively inviolable. In taking his immovable stands against the scientific theories of his day—in a few flicks of his "thought experiments," he demolished the then-reigning concepts of the ether and absolute space-time—Einstein serves as a shining example of the moral strength of those who are guided by intuitive truth and values. They express these values by taking principled stands and courageous actions. Although typically they are neither rigid nor stubborn, their testimony is not for hire. If everyone has a price, theirs cannot be measured in material terms or social rewards. They have discovered something to believe in and to live by that exceeds their need to survive on any terms. Living such a life, a life unswervingly guided by realizing the value of who we are and what we are a part of—Life, Humanity, the Cosmos—this is the highest form of mental health. It is exemplified by our greatest heroes:

Jefferson, Lincoln, Gandhi, Einstein, Mandela, Sakharov, and King, who incidentally may not always have deserved the highest marks in the nickel-and-dime morality of everyday social and sexual relationships.

Anatomy of the Psyche

The foundation on which the recognition of spiritual value rests is the truth that each of us, beyond the conscious ego, has a unique core being, the spiritual unconscious, which must be uncovered and developed, step-by-step and day-by-day. Out of this core being springs our core spiritual values, living by which gives us our unique meaning and purpose.

The ego is our conscious awareness and material will; it perceives external reality and reconciles it with internal drives and makes plans and takes actions that work to satisfy our material and survival needs. Metaphorically, it sits atop a well that plunges below the surface of consciousness to dip through the layers of the Freudian and spiritual unconscious to connect with the soul-giving water table that we all draw nourishment from: the underground stream of Spirit. The ego is characterized as self-centered or egotistical because its ultimate concern is with individual survival and achievement—not the good of all. Whatever altruism it manifests comes out of self-interest. Through its agency, we try to treat others well not because of their intrinsic value, but to court their assistance in achieving our individual goals and in perpetuating our "selfish genes" and inclusive fitness.

In marked contrast, the spiritual unconscious, typically and initially lying outside of awareness, can have a growing influence on the conscious ego. As the repository of higher values that transcend the interests of the egocentric self, it can influence the ego to behave altruistically. And through its connection to Spirit—called variously the ground of being, the universal Self, Mind, or Will, also related, however tenuously, to the collective unconscious of Jung's psychology and the God of mainstream religions—the spiritual unconscious potentially has access to the united minds of all conscious beings and can draw on the vital energy locked up in the mass of the material world.

As the spiritual unconscious becomes increasingly conscious, we develop a spiritual self whose faculties of intuition and empathy give us the added awareness to experience our connection to all-consciousness, to become united with Spirit. For the self connected and infused with Spirit, altruism is no indirect way to self-aggrandizement but is the very essence of having a soul and its awareness that we are all constituents of one higher Self. Each individual self is connected to all others and is a reflection of the totality of the higher Self, just as each constituent cell of a tissue or organ is connected to all others and to the whole as a microcosm, what I call a spiritual hologram, a part that has the fundamental qualities of the whole in miniature, limited form. (It is a supreme irony that becoming conscious of the spiritual sources of creativity may lead to self-consciousness in artists and musicians and therefore work against that very creativity. Maybe Wittgenstein had something worthwhile to say on this issue: analytic therapists should remain silent about the unconscious sources of the works of real artists.)

In this scheme, the Freudian unconscious—the unconscious repressed—is the repository only of repressed (and dissociated?) egocentric drives and conflicts and therefore is conceptually distinct from the spiritual unconscious. The latter's presumed connection to forces and structures that lie outside individual experience—as examples, the deep structures of spatiotemporal causality, the frameworks for the acquisition of language and the moral sense—is one of the fundamental differences between Freudian and Jungian theory and between the psychological and the spiritual perspectives. On this account, the spiritual self possesses knowledge, largely unconscious, without the empirical experience to account for it, by way of its connection to Spirit. In Freudian theory, the contents of the unconscious are almost entirely limited to the experiences of conflicts between drives and controls that have been repressed, for in this theory the individual mind has access to no other minds and other universes, only to the empirical world provided by the testimony of the senses. Moreover, all memories reside within individual minds—they are not stored in racial memory nets or in any other possible fields that connect individual minds together to form a larger whole, as theorists such as Rupert Sheldrake propose.[30] As opposed to such field theories, according to Freudian theory, individuals can have no knowledge of the cosmos—knowledge that could possibly transcend the "subject-object split"—except what is given by the data of the five senses.

From the vantage point of this schema, spiritual therapy aims for no lesser achievement than gaining access to the true spiritual self, becoming aware of its values, and developing the character strength to act on them persistently. Therapeutic success ultimately derives from opening the channel between the spiritual self and the universal Self, which I call Spirit, whose energy and truth might inspire and enlighten the conscious ego. In the process the individual comes to know other minds and to recognize that ideas of separateness pertaining to the empirical world of people and things are illusions, albeit necessary and useful ones for purposes of biological survival and achievement.

The Decontamination of Spirituality

Informed by this picture, we are now in a position to reframe Freud's critique of religion and spirituality. By pointing to the irrationality and infantile neediness of many forms of spiritual belief, particularly in the existence of an interpersonal, anthropomorphic God-figure, Freud was calling attention to its contamination by neurosis and psychosis and by arrests in psychobiological development. If, however, we can offer spirituality cleansed of these contaminants, then the psychodynamic therapies, along with biological, interpersonal and behavioral techniques, become purifying early steps on the path to a healthy spiritual life. These steps involve repairing the conscious ego and its will with all the effective techniques at our command. In so doing, we reduce the severity of symptoms, undo the effects of arrested emotional and cognitive development, and enhance more mature attitudes and behavior. We accomplish these tasks by the appropriate use of medication, psychological insight, cognitive-behavioral relearning, and spiritual modes of repair, such as meditation, prayer, yoga, and creative visualization. In the process, we free the individual self to become spiritual on healthy terms, not by adopting obsessive-compulsive rituals and worshiping concrete anthropomorphic figures of spiritual agency, the handiwork of an overburdened constricted ego, but by gaining suprapersonal awareness of the whole Self and its all-inclusive universe.

Therefore, relief of symptoms and repair of faulty past learning are not competing or incidental goals in the spiritual project but the necessary means of freeing the will to attain the ultimate goal. To be successful in this venture, the patient may first have to overcome, as much as possible and typically with the help of treatment, the disastrous effects of faulty genetics and traumatic life experiences.

Appropriate Goals

Are finding the true self and realizing some of its intrinsic core values appropriate goals of psychiatric treatment? Certainly not for a psychiatry conceived purely as applied science, as a nondirective and "objective" undertaking. But for a psychiatry that is both art and science, that strives for both knowledge *and* wisdom, there can be no justification for withholding the technical expertise and spiritual guidance informed by high ideals that inspire us to reach the goals of the true and better self.

The Spiritual Terms

In the spiritual realm, "will," "belief," and "purpose" become all-important terms. Equally meaningful are "integrity," "value," and "identity." In contrast to their scientific, empirical counterparts—cause, effect, technique, and mechanism and similarly, instinct, drive, reflex, ego control, and social class—these spiritual terms introduce forms of meaning and influence that are essentially supra-causal and, therefore, outside the boundaries of normal science. The difference can be put simply: spiritual truth aims at telling us what is ultimately worth believing and doing, what we ought to do, and what we can hope for; ordinary science tells us *how* to do it and why people believe what they do and what effects these beliefs have on individual and social behavior, on the individual and society. For instance, any supposedly scientific claim that one race is genetically inferior to another in terms of intelligence is neither worth believing nor worth acting on until repeated studies controlled for bias support it *and* the means to correct or compensate for the alleged inequity can be made available. For moral-spiritual reasons, a ready acceptance of such a hurtful finding must be firmly resisted. Determining the many reasons that people would come to believe such a claim and to generate "supportive data" and thereby contribute to the stigma of those labeled would, of course, be a legitimate subject of scientific inquiry.

Science is the discovery of lawful patterns of means, causes, and consequences; spirituality involves, as a consequence of our connection to a higher Self, the intuition of ultimate ends and the will to work toward achieving them. It would be foolish and, indeed, has been historically disastrous to try to get along with only one of these forms of truth. The resulting rotten fruits range from the trivialities of Skinner boxes to the horrors of the gas chambers.

Spirituality and Mental Health

From the spiritual viewpoint, mental health and disorder always go beyond chemical imbalances, psychological mechanisms, and social conditions to deal with the consequences of being true to oneself or not, of having a soul or snuffing it out, of maintaining integrity or losing it. Looked at in this way, mental heath is a form of spiritual wholeness. The most meaningful aspect of emotional disorder, the part attesting to a loss of meaning and purpose, derives from a miscarriage of spirituality, from a maiming of the soul, which may lead to the development of a false or hollow self with deficient values. The implications are clear: the repair of the damaged or lost soul requires an influx of healing values and ideals as personified by caring individuals of sound judgment who serve as role models, mentors, and spiritual therapists. This is a true moral therapy, and it cannot be conveyed solely by effective medicines or psychological relearning apart from the goodwill and integrity of those who offer these healing inspirations. What these discontented souls need is not another explanation but a heightened experience, not a psychological insight but a spiritual awakening.

What should not be surprising then is that patients keep searching for answers even after having already undergone years of work with well-credentialed therapists. They have been given appropriate medicine and good insight into the causes of their discontent, but having failed to connect spiritually with clinicians who manifest uplifting values, they still feel untethered and demoralized. No longer severely symptomatic or plagued by self-defeating patterns of behavior, they still lack true contentment and the sense of purpose that comes from finding and living a calling. In contrast, when they feel truly appreciated—for their fine personal qualities, for their courage and persistence, for the survival of their soul against all odds, in short, for their special moral-spiritual qualities—only then do they make the spiritual connection that fills them with meaning and that inspires and strengthens them to climb the steep path of spiritual growth.

What I am saying is that the practice of psychiatry and psychotherapy that aspires to be more than a medical specialty or a psychological technique, that has the courage to become a true healing art and science, is forced to acknowledge that human beings must find appropriate values to believe in and live by, taking account of who we truly are and what we realistically have the potential to become. This is the great journey of the human soul: finding and developing the true self, living it in a calling, and arriving at a state of feeling blessed to be alive in a meaningful world.

The True Self and Identity

The nature of identity is, of course, one of the great conundrums at the interface of philosophy and psychology, and we cannot claim to have illuminated its deepest secrets or dispelled its mysteries. But we do know that we all have a focal point of experience located somewhere (really nowhere) behind our eyes and in our bodies and that it is connected in some mysterious way to our material existence, but that even though it has a certain constancy over time, it does not entirely reside in the spatiotemporal world. Yet our sense of it is obliterated when a certain mass of our brain cells is rendered dysfunctional. We do not know whether our personal identity survives biological death, a source of great angst to many, although the survival of the soul is an article of faith in most of the great religions. But we do know that the sense of self is stronger in some than in others and that those who have the strongest sense of identity tend to be courageous and steadfast in their commitments, the hallmarks of strong character.

Another way of putting this is that individuals with a strong sense of self have a strong, unbroken will, which usually cannot be compromised, although a pretended show of submission may function as a strategic retreat. Viktor Frankl's discovery of his inviolable self amid the degradations of a concentration camp, which he credits for his physical survival, is the subject of one of the most arresting descriptions of the power and indestructibility of identity in modern literature.[31]

Individuals with a weak sense of self have typically had their will split, broken, or arrested in development by overpowering forces in the environment. Otto Rank claimed that this breaking, which he judged to be a major source of neurosis, also serves the protective function, like a circuit breaker, of keeping the soul's spirit or creative spark alive.[32] He went on to call the neurotic a failed artist who could become creative again by repairing the broken artistic will. This is another take on our idea of dissociative splitting as defense against shattering of the self that defines psychosis, the subject of chapter 5.

The False Self

There are three main downsides to splitting: the first is the overall weakening effect on character of a fractured self; second, but less obvious, is that a split-off internal saboteur is likely to result, and this saboteur works to thwart our most cherished hopes for success; and third, in its place, a fabricated, false self often emerges to compensate for the loss of integrity of the true self. This false self might speak in a high-born English accent, hiding the individual's rural Mississippi origins. Or it might invent the pedigree of a Latvian-Jewish survivor of Auschwitz despite having never left his native Switzerland during World War II. This latter hoax was actually perpetrated by the infamous B. Wilkomirski, who hid his true origins for years and caused untold embarrassment to his unwitting sponsors.[33]

Less extreme versions involve individuals who hide their ethnic origins out of shame or social ambition or who disguise their base intentions by assuming a façade of general bonhomie. The truly hollow are the con artists who never reveal their true feelings, not even to themselves, but who can be counted on to try to ingratiate themselves with all whom they see as exploitable.

The detection of a false self is at first a matter of intuition, empirically confirmed by experiences of blustering affect and flip inconsistency of views, witnessed depressingly often in candidates for political office. We sense that the candidates are inauthentic: too glib or nice to be genuine, making claims of good works as a cover for overweening narcissism and a sense of entitlement. The intense media exposure of political campaigns is often thought to do best at differentiating the candidates as to the virtues of their specific programs for change. But because their handlers may teach them how to spin their positions to gloss over points of controversy, voters are easily led astray, a discovery often made too late to undo the resulting social damage of incompetent winners of elections. Media exposure may do better, at least to the attuned observer, at ferreting out inauthenticity of self because ultimately we cannot fail to communicate our integrity or its lack by the way we present ourselves. The costs of being tone-deaf to these matters are incalculable. But pandering candidates who speak in the hollow, orotund tones of sanctimonious conviction as they abandon old positions like unfashionable clothing and who make revelatory slips of contemptuous attitudes toward "the lower classes" fatally compromise their chances of winning office.

In many cases, the will of the people would seem to favor a candidate of doubtful competence with a well-defined identity and black-and-white morals over an intelligent advocate of more nuanced positions who does not seem comfortable in his own skin. Needless to say, such outcomes do not always augur well for the community. After all, strong character, despite its intrinsic value, does not ensure good leadership because charisma and specialized administrative and technical skills may also be required. But it becomes a hugely negative quality when it is accompanied by rigidity, self-righteousness, and the inability to admit and learn from mistakes. When these qualities are added, character should no longer be called strong, but rather rigid and regressive.

Race, Sexuality, and Identity

The arenas in which identity has played out most dramatically in our time are race and sexuality. With the election of the first African American president in the United States in 2008, the culmination of years of struggle for racial equality, African-Americans have become remarkably prouder and more comfortable with this aspect of their identity. Similarly, with the outlawing of the "Don't Ask, Don't Tell" requirement for gay Americans to serve in the military and the legal acceptance of same-sex marriage in many states, out-of-the-closet homosexuality has also become less stigmatized and therefore more openly embraced as a vital element of identity. These count as great moral-spiritual developments in our society since they implicitly recognize that race and sexual identity have nothing to do with the moral worth of an individual or social group. Yet how one comes to terms with one's identity does make a difference. Hiding one's ethnic origins or sexual orientation in the service of personal ambition or avoidance of public embarrassment does compromise character. Iconic public figures who deny the facts or feign ignorance when they are outed as gay or of Jewish or African descent do themselves no favors by so forfeiting their moral integrity. Trying to sever connections to a persecuted minority, as many assimilated Jews did in both pre- and post-Nazi Germany, does not typically attest to good character and tends to overlook, sometimes necessarily for purposes of survival, the harmful consequences to the self and to the quality of personal relationships that might ensue.

Values and Careers

Beyond affirming our true ethnicity and biopsychological gender, we must also resist environmental pressures to affirm moral and political positions and choose socially acceptable careers that go against our essential nature. Exhibiting racial prejudice and approving persecution of minorities or choosing a profession purely for status or money is antithetical to leading a spiritual life, which is intimately bound up with authenticity and inclusiveness. We must do what our essential nature dictates, from the way we materially adorn our lives to how we choose our work. And we must not devalue anyone simply on the basis of their race, religion, or color. Leading an authentic life inspired by the high ideals given by spiritual awareness is one of the prime goals of a spiritual therapy. Undoing anti-spiritual attitudes, such as racial prejudice and crass materialism, is the inevitable consequence of finding and developing the true self, another definition of therapeutic success in spiritual terms. Taking these steps makes it ever more likely that we will also find our true calling and a state of blessedness.

Identity Formation

We are indebted to Erik Erikson[34] for elucidating the role of early identifications and the later modifications of these early identifications in forming the enduring qualities of a defined self. During adolescence, in particular, the developing person has the task of sorting out those parental attributes that fit with his or her true nature and those that go against it, identifying with the former, rejecting the latter, or transforming both to make for better fits with both the true self and the real environment. The "self psychologists," primarily Kohut[35] and his followers, also outlined the disastrous consequences for identity of witnessing the destruction of one's parents as role models, who are the personified ideals toward which children naturally strive. When parents are convicted for criminal or immoral behavior or excommunicated from church or society, as the Nazis did to Jewish and other ethnic minorities, such degradations of ego ideals are disastrous for a young person's sense of identity and his or her ability to forge a successful career and find a calling. Perhaps even more damaging are nasty divorces in which one parent effectively brainwashes the children, as in parental alienation syndromes, to believe that the other parent is evil or worthless and no longer a fit person to emulate. Undoing these effects, if at all possible, is certain to keep lawyers, judges, therapists, and deprogrammers busy for the foreseeable future.

Attaining Spirituality

Even though the meaning of spirituality has been contaminated in our time by fundamentalist religion and New Age pieties, I have been trying to rescue its essential meaning, which is the state of being in touch and melding with a higher consciousness that encompasses all individual "loci" of consciousness and thereby constitutes all-consciousness. We recognize that there is a whole that is larger than each of us. This higher consciousness is, or has as its content, the energized spirit of reality that lies ordinarily out of awareness behind the world of appearances. Spirit is a force or energy, variously termed the life force, the common will, the universal consciousness, or the thing-in-itself.[36] It cannot be perceived directly by our ordinary five senses but rather is revealed to our spiritual self by a special faculty of suprasensible knowing. We usually call this faculty intuition, but other terms have been commonly used, such as the sixth sense, inspiration, and heightened awareness.

We are not disturbed when artists and composers allude to this form of knowing as the source of their best works, but doubts arise when it is suggested that we everyday people can share in its awareness, especially when the major reductionistic belief systems of modern times have denied its very existence. But every time we are moved by a profoundly beautiful piece of music or art, by the awesome glory of nature or by an inspiring example of moral behavior—manifesting in a Mandela, Sakharov, or Lincoln world-altering forms of wisdom and generosity—we become touched by Spirit and experience its emanations in the empirical world and in our own souls. The same is true when we empathize with the sufferings of those whom misfortune has struck, when we realize that "no man is an island," that we share a common self and a common fate. Besides these spontaneous encounters with Spirit, there are age-old practices that heighten awareness and allow us to work toward communing with the spiritual ground of being. These disciplined forms of meditation, visualization, prayer, yoga, chanting, and physical bowing and whirling, the last typically associated with Sufism, all play a major role in the great religions, occupying their common spiritual core.

Spirit itself, the object of this heightened awareness, is also known by many other names: the higher power, the organizing principle, the universal self, the life force, God, divine love, Buddha, Dao, the gods, our better angels, fate and destiny. Although many of these terms have specific metaphysical or theological implications, their common agency is the activation of the human will to feats of creativity and healing. This activation comes with discovering our spiritual self and projecting its will into the world. When this is done, when we resolve to stand up for our true self, then Spirit can enter our life and reveal to us what is good and healing. It imbues us with the faith and will to lead a good life, to living right.

Emphasis on Mental Health

Since this is a book about psychiatry and mental health, I place most emphasis on that aspect of spirituality involved in activating and strengthening the will to health. But understand that the creative and healing will takes many forms: the higher will to life, to health, to faith, to knowledge, to social repair, to love, even to wealth in the broadest sense. The specific form it takes may be determined by the human context that calls it forth. But in any context, the Spirit, through its instrumental arm, the Will, is active, seeking, directive, shaping. It never merely reflects *what is* but actively determines *what ought to be*. It has no truck with negativity and therefore avoids unbalanced prophets of doom. In an important sense, the will creates its own truth, and therefore, truth is to some extent created by human beings in action, within the constraints imposed by the structures of empirical reality. Accepting these constraints, such as the inevitability of biological death, is a crucial difference between being spiritual and becoming psychotic.

Chapter 4
THE WILL: ITS PARALYSIS AND ACTIVATION

Summary. After a case illustration, I describe the phenomena of paralysis of the will. Severe depression, as the most common substrate, comes in for extended discussion. Other common causes of such paralysis are phobic fears and, most important of all, a split-off internal saboteur, discussed further in the next chapter. The repair of a blocked will, although dependent on medical and psychological interventions, often requires an infusion of spiritual values, typically provided by the care and guidance of a spiritual therapist and group who exemplify a commanding purpose for taking resolute action. In an attempt to become a "respectable" applied science, conventional psychotherapy excised the "will" concept from its operational terms and, in the process, marginalized the spiritual factors dependent on it, such as character strength, moral responsibility, and moral treatment. Trying to make do without value-laden terms such as "character disorders" and "character flaws," instead substituting more seemingly value-free diagnoses such as personality disorders, has left the field in a confused and weakened state, in which these behavioral pattern disorders are found to be confusingly overlapping and refractory to treatment. Looking at the task from a spiritual perspective, we are in a position to rescue spirituality from Freud's rejection of spiritual experience. By recognizing the spiritual dimension of human motivation, we gain a better understanding of what it means to have a free will and to be held morally responsible. The development of the will in the course of psychological development is briefly examined. From the humble beginnings of curbing our egocentric needs, we develop a majestic power—creative and healing free will—capable of overcoming the mood disorders and the character flaws that formerly blocked it.

The Case of Doreen

Doreen was in her fourteenth year of graduate school, lacking only the dissertation to complete her PhD in sociology. She had already successfully passed the preliminary exams and done the research supporting her thesis. On repeated occasions her advisor had offered to help write up the results so that she could get the degree and career she deserved. She had declined all such offers. Each year for the past dozen or so years, she had registered and paid the fees to retain her pre-doctoral status. In therapy, she affirmed her good intentions, but they were waylaid by bouts of depression, anxiety, a sense of fragmentation, noisy neighbors, and romantic breakups. Each of these issues was treated from a combined biomedical and psychosocial perspective, so that by the end of her third year of treatment, she was virtually free of symptoms but still unable to complete her written thesis or to allow anyone else to help her do it.

Turning to the psychological meanings of her block, we uncovered that her father had been let go from his untenured position in the local university's sociology department when Doreen was around eight or nine. The impact on the family was catastrophic. Her father began drinking heavily and became psychotically depressed and physically abusive toward his wife and Doreen, who had previously been his special favorite and "male heir." Her conscious goal in the present was to restore the family's honor by becoming an academic success in a way that was denied her father. Yet she also was aware of hateful as well as adoring feelings toward him and guilt for displacing her mother, once beautiful and treasured and now functioning as family servant. In addition, she harbored hateful feelings toward the academic establishment for its life-ruining treatment of her father. Thus, she was obviously ambivalent about earning a doctorate in sociology, so bound up with the failure of her father as an academic and the field that she judged to be responsible for his failure. And as is often the case in such blocks, success also carried the symbolic meaning of a forbidden oedipal victory, magnified by her becoming identified with her father's fate and her attempted restitution of his stature. She felt it would be a betrayal of his memory (and her mother) to succeed at a task so tainted with loss and betrayal.

Yet none of these insights and approaches got her any closer to finishing her doctorate. Relieved of her anxiety, depression, and phobic fears, and having gained insight into her psychological conflicts, she still took no further steps to write her dissertation. As one of my colleagues put it, "her unconscious had her by the throat." Instead of moving forward, she abruptly proclaimed a total loss of interest in the project. As we began to marshal evidence for the existence of an internal saboteur blocking her progress (the subject of the next chapter and a dynamic I was just beginning to appreciate), she became increasingly uncomfortable and emotionally remote and then abruptly terminated both her individual and group treatment, in the process pointing out my many faults and those of her fellow group members. When last heard from, she had withdrawn from her doctoral program and taken a job as an administrator for a private research organization.

This case represents a common story of blockage of the will due to paralyzing phobic anxiety and depression and psycho-moral conflicts, such as honoring her father's memory versus succeeding at the academic game that he had so ruinously lost and that she despised. Looking ahead, it also demonstrates how my failure to deal in a timely fashion with her split-off internal saboteur led to a treatment failure. For therapists to review such failures, especially with patients who have uncommon potential for success, is, to say the least, painfully humbling. Redeeming such situations is best done by regarding them not as failures but as the result of misconceptions in need of future correction. This requires an abject admission: not infrequently, we therapists are initially overmatched by powerfully destructive forces that inhabit our patients' lives. In the next chapter, I hope to demonstrate how deviously powerful an internal saboteur can be and how much groundwork must be done to put the patient-therapist alliance in position to corral it and overcome its workings.

My unsuccessful treatment in this case resulted from two misconceptions. The first, as already mentioned, derived from initially regarding her will disorder as the consequence of depression and psychological conflict rather than also stemming from a split-off internal saboteur that needed to be neutralized. The case was lost by the time I got around to addressing this factor. The second misconception was that I could get away with assuming a stance of relative moral neutrality in confronting her failure to complete her doctorate. She lacked the moral resolve to overcome her dissociated and repressed will, and I failed to stand for the inspiring values that she needed and should have expected from a mentoring therapist. I did not point out the betrayals of trust, the cowardice, and the need for retribution manifested in her slacking off from meeting her responsibilities. In going over her case file, I found other examples of moral evasion or insensitivity on my part—for example, I did not adequately mourn with her when her mother died—all of which contributed to her loss of faith in me as the moral force she desperately needed to complete her professional studies under duress or to abandon them for justifiable reasons. In what follows, I further the discussion of legitimizing the play of moral and spiritual values in doing effective treatment with patients such as Doreen: patients who have character flaws.

Character Flaws

Innumerable problems arise in treating patients with self-defeating personality patterns. Most of them spring from the fact that the patients have a corrupted will that works tirelessly against potentially effective steps to make repairs. When these obstructions involve repeated, often unconscious attempts to harm not only themselves but also family, friends, and colleagues, we say they have character flaws. In applying this term to patients, we are implicitly saying that they have an immoral, destructive component of their will—in Doreen's case, illustrated by betraying the commitment and trust of her university, thesis advisor, therapist and fellow group patients. In contrast, the healthy intact will is a moral-spiritual agency, a spiritual conscience, empowered not only by instincts and reflexes but also by purposeful and beneficent values and ideals. To repair the dissociated will, therefore, the true self must be strengthened by higher purposes, often personified by a therapist-mentor and a group with an aggregate will, to overcome patterns of self-defeat and harm to others.

The recognition does not come easily. Scientific empiricists, with the public esteem typically accorded to reductionists, have banished the Will from the roster of legitimate personal agencies, thereby contributing to a void in our understanding and methodology for treating character flaws. Trying to reduce character disorders to personality disorders, as most recent editions of the APA *Diagnostic and Statistical Manual* have attempted to do, is a disingenuous effort to hide the moral judgments involved in diagnosing patients as having flaws of character structure. The failure to recognize this fact explains several other failures in our understanding and treatment of these disorders, particularly why they overlap so greatly and why they are considered nearly impossible to repair, often solely attributed to a lack of "observing ego" in the patient to the exclusion of the vastly more important lacks of the moral intuition, moral resolve, and moral guidance of therapist and patient combined.

Moral disorders come in a few defined forms, such as patterns of harming, deceiving, and coercing others and, of course, oneself. The treatment they require, beyond the interventions of the criminal justice system, is moral treatment—that is, a spiritual treatment that goes beyond biomedical and psychosocial techniques to take account of the activating power of spiritual values and the paralyzing, corrupting effects of false and conflicting values.

Misconceived Science

Who and what drove psychiatrists and psychotherapists—healers of the soul—to go so far off-track? Who sold them on the idea that theirs was solely an applied science rather than a work that was only partly based on empirical science? The most meaningful part is, and always has been, a spiritual art form involving the right kind of caring attention and guidance. The impetus for providing this attention and guidance—indeed the ability to do so—comes to us from a realm of caring beyond the spatiotemporal material world and the scientific body of knowledge. To be sure, psychotherapy as an applied science serves a basic instrumental role in good treatment—but hardly the most significant role.

The hard-science followers of William of Occam, starting with the British empiricists (e.g., Locke and Hume), gained such dominance over seekers of nonempirical truth that by the twentieth century, the existence of the individual will, the human spiritual force par excellence, had been diagnosed by leading philosophers of science as an excisable wart on the body of knowledge. Behaviorists, neuroscientists, and with few exceptions mainstream psychologists had all dispensed with the concept of will to account for the initiation of human action. In almost every case its more respectable replacements were conditioned reflexes and biological drives such as sexual and aggressive instincts, with a nodding acceptance of "executive ego." Among the scientific elite, the will was not a respectable subject for discussion.[37]

In truth, the will and its phenomena do not fit within the framework of empirical science where there is no assigned place for purpose, where instead causes and effects are linked together in long, interacting mechanical chains like intersecting rows of toppling dominoes. Willful actions by definition involve nonmechanistic purposes. Ego functions, instincts, psychic determinism, classical and operant conditioning, cortical evoked potentials—these are concepts more consonant with the scientific framework. The human will, in contrast, clearly lies outside materialistic causal chains, intervening in them like bolts of lightning from the heavens. It's not that we cannot discover biological and psychological determinants of these unexpected blips of behavior. To be sure, chemical and physiological events can be correlated with many of our acts of willing, just as events in our past histories can be seen to condition us to take certain courses of action rather than others. But we are typically reduced to making these connections after the fact, after the dramas have already played out. In the lab, we see brain activity accompanying acts of will, but we do not know how they are connected, any more than we understand the mind—body connection in general. There is a fundamental incompleteness to our scientific knowledge because some of the variables lie outside the empirical world of controlled, repeatable observations and cannot be invariantly connected to them.

The practical takeaway is that we cannot always predict future events no matter how much knowledge we have of the past and present. And this is true in principle, not just in fact. Hard scientists might say that this inability, as may be the case in some instances of faulty weather forecasting, is evidence only of the incompleteness of our empirical knowledge, not the workings of chance or an illusory, supra-causal force like the eruption of a spontaneous act of a free will, unnecessarily invoked to account for our lack of prior knowledge. Yet if we take account of some major changes in mathematics and physics during the twentieth century, we are not so likely to be satisfied with this conclusion. For example, Heisenberg's uncertainty principle, in accounting for the unexpected effects of the observer's act of observing on empirical phenomena, and Gödel's proof of the *incompletability*, not just incompleteness, of predictive knowledge,[38] taken together open the door to the occurrence of events outside the realm of a material causal order. As a consequence, confounding agencies such as creative spontaneity and free will, not just the workings of chance, become more acceptable realities in modern thought, not only to the mystically spiritual but to the respectably scientific as well. To be sure, the undetermined phenomena of quantum micro-events bear only a suggestive relationship to the acausal willful actions of human macro-behavior. But there is no overlooking the paradigm shift away from strict determinism once we recognize that the spatiotemporal universe is not the only possible universe and, more importantly, not the only universe to which we might possibly gain access. Otherwise, string theory and other theories that postulate multiple dimensions and universes are pure nonsense.

Why shouldn't we throw them into the wastebasket of all theories based on so-called ghosts in the world machine, as strict empiricists from the past would have us do?

The Free Purposeful Will

But what exactly are we claiming when we say free will exists?[39] The dictionary definition of will is a "faculty of the mind that . . . determines action and esp. moral action in accordance with ideals, principles, and facts . . . as distinguished from instinctive or purely natural desires."[40] On this account, the problem for science becomes immediately apparent. The will is not an instinctual or natural psychobiological instigator of action but rather a moral-spiritual agency spurred on by ideals and values, at best refined by critical thinking, but not strictly determined by empirical facts. Like electrons that abruptly jump from one orbit to another and show general indeterminacy of location or velocity per quantum physics, there is a seemingly spontaneous agency at play here. More meaningfully, moral scruples or intuitive solutions pop into our heads and influence our thinking and behaving, and these intuitive leaps typically link and often subordinate our natural survival and pleasure-seeking drives to higher purposes, such as keeping our promises and loyalties and trying to repair the world. The wonder is that, by acts of will, we can sometimes divert the demands of our self-centered, comfort-seeking needs to take steps that confer no immediate material benefits on us as individuals or members of groups. Rather, we take these actions for the purpose of promoting the ideals of higher, spiritual beings, which typically involve caring generosity toward others, among whom are living beings we neither know nor can directly connect to our own material well-being but whom we somehow recognize as fellow creatures who share with us a common soul. In fact, having a soul means that we recognize we are parts of a common whole, and this membership obliges us to take care, be loyal, and feel gratitude, not just to kin and clan, but to the whole cosmos.

These considerations lead us to conclude that in the absence of the existence of a will free to override human instincts and reflexes, there can be no moral responsibility and no spiritual therapy. Spiritual therapy presupposes acts of transcendence that go beyond satisfying not only egocentric needs but also the entire universe of spatiotemporal determinants of behavior. Only a free will inspired by intuited transcendent values can take such actions purposefully. Furthermore, without free will, we cease to be moral-spiritual agents. Assigning moral responsibility in the absence of real choice is absurd. In the field of forensic psychiatry, wrongdoers are typically absolved of responsibility if they do not know right from wrong when they commit a crime or if the impulse to do it is irresistible. None of us should be held accountable for actions that we *had* to perform, that we were coerced into doing by external or internal forces belonging to the realm of spatiotemporal causality. And of course, in the spatiotemporal scientific universe, there are no other kinds of human actions. But in the spiritual realm intuited values and strong character, over and above social learning and strictly enforced laws, allow us to override the causal determinants of bad behavior to do the good, just as weak character and poor moral judgment offer insufficient resistance to giving in to our worst impulses.

As deterministic scientists, we have no business blaming, much less punishing, people for behaving badly. From the empirical scientific perspective, all their misbehaviors, from minor theft to first-degree murder, are causally determined. People have to do what they do. We would be justified only in confining bad actors, not punishing them, to prevent them from doing further harm. (I will take up this theme again in Chapter 7). Yet without disavowing the implications of science, we as a society do blame and punish misbehaving criminals. How do we justify these contradictory practices of the criminal justice system? Obviously, by appealing to a moral code, a set of universal values that inform society's laws, which we judge to have been knowingly and voluntarily violated by those we condemn and punish. But as objective scientists, we are not entitled to make these moral condemnations because every event in the empirical world, notwithstanding the tenets of quantum physics, is conceived to be strictly determined.

Fortunately, this deterministic theory is recognized to be inadequate, and even more thankfully, the criminal justice system and society in general don't buy it. Rather, the societal norm is that some illegal and immoral behaviors are freely and knowingly done, whereas others are not. Ideally only the perpetrators of the first are held accountable and brought to justice. Others are judged to have diminished responsibility as a result of mental or physical impairment or various forms of coercion. Consider the threat to a bank officer, "Get me the access codes to all your bank's accounts; otherwise your son will be killed." Since such dire threats sometimes lead to criminal behavior as the perceived best outcome, the severity of the judicial verdict is likely to be diminished considerably because of the nature of the threat.

The crucial determinants of a judge's or jury's verdicts in these cases involve their judgments as to how much freedom the perpetrator had to pursue an alternative course of action to avoid committing the crime.

We must try to differentiate more clearly between the coerced and the merely inclined, persuaded or seduced. We might then be in a position to show how to achieve true freedom by means of an effective spiritual therapy. In the process, we can hopefully better distinguish those who deserve punishment from those who do not.

Species Limits on Free Will and Responsibility

Although beings other than humans, such as our pet dogs, cats, and horses, give evidence of a rudimentary will, we do not usually accord them the degree of choice that would make them morally responsible, even when they appear to act responsibly, as when family dogs protect us from intruders or don't retaliate after children stick pencils into their ears. We eventually come around to postulating that their seeming choices are, in fact, part of their DNA and the results of instinctive and conditioned reflexes. We say that wolves who abruptly stop short of ripping out the throats of their fellow wolves are not exercising free will but are acting from that class of instincts termed "anti-instincts." In any case, we do not usually regard these nonhuman animals as moral agents, no matter how much we might love our dogs for their apparent human-like qualities.

For example, our Samoyed Mooshka, friendly to humans but wolf-like toward other creatures, had the habit of prying open the refrigerator to devour the prime rib roast we were all looking forward to eating for dinner. After a few unsuccessful attempts at scolding and otherwise conditioning behavior change, we concluded that Mooshka was hard-wired to be carnivorous whenever the opportunity presented, a fact best dealt with by storing meat out of his reach. But when our adolescent son wolfed down a chocolate cake that we were saving for dessert, he was reprimanded for his inconsiderate behavior and expected to do better in the future. He was held responsible for his actions and also given the message that his pleasure principle needed to become more principled, not just dialed down by punitive conditioning.

Our premise was that our son, like all human beings at their best, possesses a morally informable will that gives him the ability to override his basic appetites. We attributed to him a free will, synonyms for which are volition and choice, as opposed to rigidly determined instinct and reflex. Of course, human beings are not always at their best. And some who are at their best may not have the mental capacity to make good moral judgments and behave accordingly. It is the task of the criminal justice system, with the help of mental health and other forensic specialists, to determine degree of innocence or guilt and whether punishment or remediation is the best sentence in these cases.

As previously indicated, choosing or judging freely, leading to consciously self-determined and noncoerced behavior, is only a possibility because we do not always have the choices we think we have. Once we recognize that our drives, motives, and strictures may lie outside awareness, we may have to admit that sometimes we do not act freely or know the real reasons behind our behavior. Every day we do things because of conditioned reflexes and covert brain spikes; out of hidden ambition, envy, and jealousy; or because we want to be approved of and cared for, all factors whose operation we tend to deny. We self-righteously claim that we are acting on principle, but we may be victims of our own biases and illusions.

Imagine the following scenario, based on an actual experience at college. A distinguished but approval-seeking philosopher is arguing that human beings are blessed with freedom of the will. Some students of B. F. Skinner, the developer of operant conditioning psychology and a strong debunker of freedom, attend the lecture to see if they can override the lecturer's apparent free will as he paces back and forth on the lecture platform. Every time he roams to the left side of the platform, they smile in apparent agreement, but when he moves to the right, they frown their disapproval. Before long the professor is giving his lecture defending freedom of the will entirely stationed at the left corner of the platform. When these phenomena are brought to his attention, he becomes flustered and defensive instead of admitting that even the best intentions can be subverted.

This possibility adds to our admiration for those who can decode ever-present subliminal influences, from the frowns of listeners to the shaky claims of TV advertising, and retain their ability to make free and rational choices. In making this judgment, we are recognizing that subliminal influences such as may occur in operant conditioning in the lab or in watching TV ads, are not coercive and therefore cannot entirely absolve us of moral responsibility. We retain some responsibility for resisting those who would cleverly convince us to choose bad products and bad courses of action.

Unconscious Motivation and Narcissistic Injury

Freud called the discovery of unconscious motivation, which limits the extent of our rational self-control, one of the three blows to man's "narcissism" that modern science has inflicted. The other two humbling discoveries are that the sun, not the earth, is the center of our world, and that instead of uniquely created beings, we are the descendents of apes. As he so often did, Freud showed uncanny brilliance in elucidating how scientific discoveries undermine human grandiosity. But his conclusions cannot be accepted uncritically. In the guise of arguing facts—such as the truth of biological evolution versus the claims of religion—he was in fact advancing a much larger value-permeated agenda about what we human beings can legitimately know and what forces truly motivate us. As a scientist of his day, Freud had a bias in favor of deterministic causality and against influential spirituality. According to him, we can legitimately learn about the effects of our drives and reflexes but not about the effects of our spiritual ideals, except as they can be reduced to biologically based psychological forces. Spiritual knowledge and influence have no substantive existence for Freud. Despite being an avid collector of ancient works of art, he confessed to having no emotional reaction to any piece of art or music. According to him, people invoke the reality of spiritual experience to rationalize their infantile needs, especially to feel special or to experience the bliss of being bathed in a universal amniotic fluid. In emphasizing apparently observable forces such as the sexual and aggressive instincts, he thought of himself as erecting a scientific bulwark against superstition and occultism.

Beyond Determinism

But the science Freud was upholding, with its emphasis on strict determinism, was already eroding at the time he was formulating his philosophy of human nature. As we mentioned before, quantum physics, particularly the work of Heisenberg and Schrödinger, introduced the idea that the observer so affects what is being observed that big gaps open up in the chains of cause and effect that were previously thought to be seamlessly linked, and in the process certainty is replaced by varying degrees of probability. After all, one of the requirements of scientific knowledge is that the influence of the observing mind be neutralized in the interests of objectivity. By the scientific method, the experimental observer is supposed to become a blank recording machine with no biases. But if the mere act of observation, irrespective of bias, changes the data, then we have to refine our notions about observable truth. This recalibration has paved the way not only for a measure of indeterminism in science but also for the play of a supra-temporal agency like will or spirit in introducing totally unpredictable elements into our lives. The result is that modern scientists find notions of unpredictability and incompletability much less threatening than did scientists of Freud's generation. Even Einstein, who more than anyone set the ball rolling for the new scientific perspective, had great trouble accepting its implications. For him, to say that observable truth was at best probable, not determined with certainty, was like saying that God was throwing dice with our lives, instead of merely leaving room for a transcendent free will to operate.[41]

The Spiritual Depths

Despite his circumscribed, culture-bound worldview, Freud made a great contribution by opening our eyes to the vast world of unconscious forces that secretly influence every aspect of our lives. It was left to some of Freud's early followers to explore the spiritual depths of these unconscious influences. Now we can entertain the possibility not only that repressed instinctual pressures— sexual, aggressive, passive-dependent—influence our overt behavior, but also that at a deeper level of the unconscious mind, spiritual forces can override these instinctual drives and reflexes. And like instincts, these forces are also part of our deep psychic structure, which means they do not have to be learned to exist, nor do they have to be repressed to be unconscious. They operate, mostly secretly and unbidden, because our brains are constructed to organize sensory experience in certain ways: for example, made up of separate objects and events located in space and time and connected in causal chains. As Chomsky argued, the human mind also has the "deep structure" to develop linguistic fluency by soaking up spoken language and ordering it syntactically. Less obviously, our brains, or rather their mental outgrowths, have the potential to operate as extrasensory receivers, with connections to a collective or spiritual consciousness that give us access to the promptings of a larger Self-Will that lies both "inside" and "outside" ourselves, in fact outside the spatiotemporal world altogether.

Otherwise, how do we ever gain the intuitive moral knowledge that, for example, the sense of racial superiority is a fascist evil, no matter what everyone around us might believe? Moreover, without such intuitive standards, how would we ever develop the character strength to oppose other widespread and harmful prejudices, particularly by overcoming their residues in ourselves from genetic wiring, early learning, and what Sheldrake has termed morphogenic fields—nongenetic repositories of racial and tribal memories, customs, and hatreds?[42] Yet Muslims, Christians, and Jews, and Africans, Caucasians, and Asians, despite their dark histories of trans-generational strife, have at times achieved mutual tolerance as fellow human beings, as they did for a time in medieval Spain and as they do now, to a greater or lesser extent, in multiethnic Western democracies.

Beyond Narcissism

In light of the possibility of nonempirical knowledge, we come up with a different take on the significance of unconscious motivation. It is only sometimes a blow to our "narcissism"—namely, when we think we are acting from the highest motives, only to discover the worms of jealousy and masochism at the core of our being. At other times our unconscious motives may be like sand in oysters, base materials that can be transformed into pearls of spiritual wisdom. If the unconscious mind contained only primitive, repressed material, then many of our unconsciously motivated actions *would* reek of rotten regression. But if the unconscious mind is an open system, connected to and permeated by Spirit and its collective goodwill (and sometimes not so good) then acting unconsciously might lead to the manifestations of a higher wisdom, identical to the creative acts of the inspired artist, healer and moral agent. Exercising conscious, rational self-control is, therefore, not always the highest good. In fact, going into the trance of inspiration could bring out the very best in us as artists and moral agents; and instead of constituting a blow to our egocentric narcissism, it might be the cure of it, because we would then realize that we are sometimes merely the media through which supra-individual forces act.

For example, having joined a group touring southern France a few years ago, my wife and I discovered that during World War II the owners of our inn had hidden many of the neighboring Jews in their cellar, obstructing their evacuation to extermination camps. When the subterfuge was discovered, the local fascist authorities descended upon the inn, killed the caretakers, and reduced the whole property to rubble. After the war, the local populace took up a collection to help rebuild the manor house. When we tried to praise the innkeepers for what they had done, they would not hear of it. "What else could we have done?" these religious Huguenots asked. They also downplayed the locals' generosity in helping them rebuild the inn: neighbors are supposed to help one another.

The innkeepers' attitude recalls those musicians and music lovers who, despite having powerful emotional responses to a composition, claim no special extra-musical meaning for it. Isn't it just good music? Beethoven's own notion that he was a channel of a higher creative agency—he claimed that his symphonies were being composed "through" him—is assigned to the realm of metaphor. Yet it is a metaphor seemingly powerful enough to convince the Irish mathematician J. W. N. Sullivan that Beethoven's music demonstrated an immense spiritual development.[43] Like everyday musicians, however, the innkeepers made no claim of a higher moral agency operating through them. But despite their humility—because of it?—we are awed by the power of their common decency.

As we turn to psychopathology, it is important to remind ourselves of these humble examples of the moral free will at work, whether consciously chosen or not. For examples of the pathologically bound will, we turn now to a discussion of depression, its most characteristic manifestation.

The Depressed Will

The syndrome of depression, as opposed to the more circumscribed feeling states of sadness and grief, can be a devastating, long-lasting disorder that burrows into every recess of mind, body, and spirit. Its victims complain of dejection and low worth, lack of energy, and loss of interest in lovemaking and other pleasurable activities. Sometimes they do not admit to feeling morose but complain more of fatigue or of various physical symptoms such as headache, back pain or problems with sleep, appetite, and bowel function. But most important of all, depressed people often cannot do the things they want to do, and at worst, they lose the will to do anything at all. Such states of paralysis are described by technical terms such as "psychomotor retardation," "mutism," and "abulia." The victims of these symptoms may not believe anything is worth doing, or they may harbor the belief, sometimes based on a delusional fear of causing irreparable harm, that they must refrain from taking any action at all.

One depressed elderly gentleman, who actually had to be catheterized, said that he did not dare urinate because he would drown everyone in town. Such a case serves to illustrate that depression is not uncommonly mixed with its opposite, manic grandiosity and psychotic delusions. It also brings home forcefully that the syndrome is meaningfully characterized as a blockage of the will. It is difficult to imagine refusing to urinate or, more commonly, refusing to eat, with such determination that tubes have to be inserted to drain urine or supply nourishment. But these are not uncommon occurrences in hospital practice. The will, paralyzed by negative ideas and impulses, has been turned against itself to impose a blockade on the biological imperative to survive, on the very will to life. In less dire circumstances, it will not let novelists write, shopkeepers sell their wares, or parents care for their children. How does the will become so blocked? In other words, how does the will become functionally depressed and therefore bound rather than free?

The Development of the Will

A review of the salient points of the development of the human will seems called for at this point. Here is a brief sketch of the process.

The infant has basic needs: to be held, cleaned, clothed, fed, and adored, needs that good parents are anxious to meet. In late infancy satisfaction of needs becomes complicated by a battle of the wills. Parents begin to insist more vigorously on social behavior: eating without smearing, gaining control of urinary and bowel functions, putting things away, and going to bed in a timely fashion. Children try to get around these curbs on their impulses. The outcome of this struggle, which determines the basic character of the individual's will in later life, is as always the product of an interaction between nature, nurture and spirit. If parents say no and impose discipline in a caring, considerate manner, often allowing the children some leeway, they will tend to accept limits without feeling violated and without being consumed with resentment over having to curb their desires. They will internalize the discipline and then be able to say no to their own immature or unrealistic wishes. Properly respected by their early caregivers, they will subsequently learn to say no to unreasonable demands made by other members of society.

The ability to say no, both to one's own problematic desires and to the persuasions of others, is what we typically call willpower.

Finally and most productively, children can be encouraged to say yes to reasonable, beneficial demands and to their own needs for self-expression. This is the beginning of becoming a cooperative person with a positive will. Such individuals can say yes wholeheartedly because they have learned and been allowed to say no first, a precondition of developing an autonomous free will. Compliance can be rendered without loss of freedom or integrity, and imagination can be given free rein without fear of losing love and identity or causing unacceptable harm to others. The rudimentary will has developed both a negative component, willpower, and a positive, productive part—the affirming, cooperative, creative faculty. Later in life, this healthy, balanced will can lead to the development of an effective work ethic that is joyous and relatively free of deadening drudgery. With increasing maturity and an ability to manage the inevitable losses of human existence, healthy individuals develop a hardheaded affirmation of the healing, creative spirit flowing through their being, a crucial condition of feeling blessed to be alive.

Further Pathologies of the Will

Miscarriages in these crucial periods of the will's development are well known because of their highly visible costs in human suffering. Phobic anxiety, a very common blocker of willful action, is typically first manifested as a fear of separation from parents that, at its most severe, can lead to school refusal. Other phobias involve fear of heights, flying, public speaking, and open or closed spaces and a terrifying aversion to insects, small animals, and sources of contamination. The phobias are now recognized as belonging on the spectrum of mood disorders, of which anxiety and depression are the common substrates.

Other common pathological syndromes of volition are passivity, oppositionalism, and impulsivity, which often come mixed together. In extreme forms of passivity, individuals take little initiative and wait for others to provide care or leadership. They are often described as obsessive worriers or simply lazy, and they tend to be complainers: things are not going well, but it is the fault of others or circumstances beyond their control. In any case they claim they can do nothing about their situation. If the situation is to be remedied, someone else or God will have to do it. If oppositionalism is added to the picture, often brought on by stifling, invasive rearing or severe neglect, those with a blocked will actively resist any suggestion, any opportunity to find solutions or to enjoy success. And they typically bite the hands that try to feed them. Would-be helpers, unless very persistent or masochistic, are soon discouraged and driven away.

For example, Lara, whose mother stayed in bed throughout her childhood, survived by developing a crust of paranoid belligerence. In the wake of a failed marriage, she was very cooperative initially, judging many of my suggestions, such as taking medications, to be helpful. But not long after she was helped to sustain a relationship and remarry, she declared herself well, stopped her mood stabilizers, and became very argumentative. When I urged her to resume medications, reminding her that prior to taking them she had been too irritable to tolerate intimacy, she became angrily resistant, claiming that I had "betrayed" her by not respecting her wishes. Lara quit therapy, and within a few years, her second husband Carl, whose treatment we discussed in Chapter Two, asked for a divorce because of her constant badgering. After initially agreeing to the terms of the property settlement, she began arguing over every detail, to the great benefit of the divorce attorneys.

Individuals who act impulsively and with paranoid belligerence tend to have the biological substrates of paranoia and bipolar mood swings, often exacerbated by invasive, permissive or inconsistent child-rearing. They often burst out of their blocked state and throw away their love, money, and goodwill in ways that lead to widespread damage to themselves and others. In striking contrast, the person with a healthy free will, including what we have previously called the will to health, *will* take every negative emotion and every unsatisfactory situation as a call to corrective action. Far from resisting advice and support, they seek it out and carefully evaluate it. Then they make decisions and act on them with determination.

As noted before, the development of a depressed, blocked, or erratic will is usually the result of combined miscarriages of nature, nurture, and spirit. From his or her biological nature, the person can be genetically predisposed to having a bound will through inheritance of the chemical and physiological substrates of mood and thought disorders: depression, manic-depression (bipolar disorder), and schizoid and paranoid tendencies, which interfere with logical thinking and formation of outside interests and connections. All these conditions can diminish the availability of energy and the ability to set clear goals, without which willful action cannot be initiated and sustained. Current scientific thinking attributes these biological deficits in part to imbalances in various neurotransmitters in the brain, such as serotonin, norepinephrine, and dopamine. These imbalances can often be corrected by effective antidepressants, mood stabilizers, and antipsychotics, but not always and not by themselves, as the following case illustrates.

The Case of Johanna

Johanna, a divorced professional woman in her fifties, had suffered from low-energy depression most of her adult life. Although able to keep a job, she had often felt like a worthless failure and had been too fatigued and lacking in motivation to get out of bed on weekends. On antidepressants such as SSRIs and SNRIs,[44] her mood improved significantly, and she became energized enough to do chores and meet with friends. Off the medicines, she slipped back into a state of lethargic paralysis. Adding one of the newer, atypical antipsychotics like Abilify to her regimen made her feel less aloof and more spontaneously interested in people and activities. Lamictal (lamotrigine), an effective remedy for bipolar depression, had an even more pronounced effect. All these medications addressed, at least to some degree, the "nature" or biomedical aspect of her blocked will.

The psychologically nurtured or learned part of Johanna's inertia can be understood as deriving from having been raised by parents who actively squashed her self-esteem and discouraged her from taking initiative or excelling. They even refused to acknowledge that she was attractive and more competent than her cognitively impaired sister. Moreover, her mother had many of the symptoms of clinical depression, qualities that were passed on to Joanna by both genetics and conditions of rearing. When Johanna was a teenager, she felt closest to her mother when they stayed up together late at night, endlessly wringing their hands over the insoluble problems facing the family. In addition to chemical imbalances, she had many longstanding conflicts and bad habits, such as inconsolably complaining instead of taking action and enjoying her successes.

Medicines may help but cannot alone overcome learned passive, oppositional, and pleasure-avoiding attitudes and behaviors. The full arsenal of psychotherapy techniques is required: insight into the sources of self-defeating patterns and the exploration of more rewarding alternatives. In Johanna's case this involved a reconstruction of her personality development, family diagnostic meetings, and willful overcoming of passive and negative patterns, such as through vigorous daily exercise and seeking out improved relationships and work opportunities. But a key to overcoming inertia, often overlooked in this and similar cases, is joining a therapeutic group capable of providing enough emotional support to bolster a flimsy personal will with inspiring ideals.

The Group Repair of the Will

The underutilization of group therapy is surely one of the most baffling phenomena of modern psychiatry and psychotherapy. Here we have an approach that, done the right way, can be vastly more efficient in terms of costs and manpower than individual therapy, yet few patients demand it, and fewer practitioners offer it. Add to this the enormous morale-boosting effect of the approach, and the mystery deepens. One suspects that the overselling of individual psychodynamic therapy for most of the twentieth century is partly to blame. During this period, young clinicians left their training and started practice somewhat familiar with two-person techniques but virtually ignorant of how to understand and manage group dynamics. The burgeoning family therapy movement, while cultivating an interest in larger social systems, diverted attention from working with potentially more available voluntary associations, as utilized in group therapy. Another crucially inhibiting factor, a topic of discussion in a later chapter, is the potential for therapeutically arranged groups to go off the rails, maximizing rather than alleviating the most primitive, maladaptive traits of member patients, perhaps to a greater extent than individual approaches.

Yet if these issues are carefully addressed, the therapeutic group has the potential for working around one of the most prevalent sources of emotional suffering: the blocked or broken will, especially in the socially isolated individual. A dawning appreciation of this possibility derived from the success of the group-based program Alcoholics Anonymous (AA) in treating addictive disorders, preeminent examples of disorders of the lonely, powerless will. What we have come to understand about the success of the AA approach—an understanding that its originators tended to dismiss—is that the weak will of the individual to resist addictive behavior is strengthened when the addict is embedded in the matrix of a supportive group will, exemplified by the AA meeting. What remains for the group therapist is to apply the example of AA, shorn of some of its anti-medical tenets, to nonaddicts also in need of volitional repair. Cases of paralytic inertia or abulia are prime candidates for this type of intervention.

Johanna Continued

Johanna had to be bounced out of an abulic state, which was not fully dispelled by medications and individual therapy. Put in a group that met weekly for two hours, she was given support and suggestions for fighting off feelings of futility and self-hatred and for taking action to overcome passive suffering. Yet for the first two years of membership, she felt so shy and uncomfortable that she could barely speak without a prepared text. As time went by and the group resisted her efforts to provoke censure and criticism, she began to tune into the fact that group members cared about her, and this led to heightened morale and interest in both group and outside activities. She was encouraged "to accentuate the positive," to stop complaining and wringing her hands, as she and her mother had "celebrated" their relationship, and instead to celebrate life by making vigorous efforts to repair her world. She began to meet regularly with Sandy (see chapter 9), one of her fellow group members, an expert in executive coaching, who, as part of their social exchange, taught her to correct major deficits in her social skills, such as responding positively when given compliments and giving warranted compliments in turn.

The effect on her relationships was dramatic. After she began to enjoy her work more and develop a network of friends on the model of group affiliation, she attributed her newfound vitality, beyond medicine, psychological insight, and behavioral practice, to group membership. She said that the group afforded her a sense of belonging, to having her own community. In addition, the coaching relationship with Sandy "breathed life" into her. She had never before felt this level of mutual identification, appreciation, and acceptance—not in family, school, or profession. Given her entrenched personality structure, however, this recognition of the group's benefits was not constant and had to be frequently reinforced. Ever sensitive to rejection and humiliation, she would from time to time deny the value of membership and have to be cajoled into staying the course. Since we are not *always* the best judges of what is good for us, we may have to be occasionally nudged, as Johanna had to be, into following an initially rejected beneficial course. Whether the nudges deliver on their promise usually becomes all too apparent over the course of time. One thing is certain: "value-free" nondirection is useless in these cases of severe mood and personality disorders. Only value-directed prescriptions, aided by group persuasion, can keep these patients on track.

Belonging

Since the sense of belonging is taken for granted by most mental health professionals, we tend not to appreciate the broad and devastating impact of its absence. What results is either an exaggerated posture of willfulness, often oppositional as in the case of Lara mentioned earlier, or a barely breathing individual will that, unsupported by the embrace of a social matrix as in the case of Johanna, can rarely act decisively and, even less, show determination in holding to a chosen course of action. Individuals who do not have intact families that dine, play, and work together or who do not belong to professional, political, and religious organizations that embody core values are vulnerable to becoming pathologically self-involved, in either inert or narcissistic modes. To compensate, they sometimes become obsessed with an external projection of a grandiosely inflated but wounded self that promises heightened esteem. The typical result is an overvalued belief system that is intolerantly absolutist, as in religious or political fundamentalism, or a freedom-escaping submission to a self-aggrandizing leader or romantic fantasy figure who embodies the isolated individual's needs for recognition and importance. To varying degrees, these needs are satisfied by various types of cults, whose appeal derives from a leadership that embodies the grandiose fantasies of the followers and repays their allegiance by offering a sense of belonging and importance. Membership in these paranoid pseudo-communities comes at a great cost, however. The members, although initially saved from their dead-end isolation, forfeit the possibility of growing a healthy, autonomous, externally directed free will with loving, healing, and creative powers.

Not just any group therapy is up to the healing task. It cannot be mainly an emotion-purging, primal-screaming, mutual-blaming verbal contact sport. Rather, the group must be a warm roast, chiding when necessary but above all else mutually caring and full of goodwill and shared joy and pain. In short, it must be a spiritual care group. What this means in practical terms and how it is brought about are the main concerns of chapters 5 and 10.

The paralyzed will of severe clinical depression and the impulsive, chaotic, or oppositional will of bipolar mood and cognitive thought disorders, the stock-in-trade of the practicing psychiatrist, often require the full gamut of medical, psychological, and spiritual approaches. To be sure, in ordinary cases of mood disturbances and phobic fears, there may be no need to deal with spiritual issues beyond giving caring attention and service and stressing the importance of manifesting these qualities in dealing with others. Yet quite frequently, there are heightened spiritual dimensions to a blocked will that require enhanced moral-spiritual treatment. We have seen this in paralytic depressions, illustrated by Johanna's case, in which the reversal of demoralization and inertia has to be sparked by envelopment in a group matrix. Similarly severe are cases of dissociative splitting, leading to the formation of an internal saboteur. The split cannot be effectively overcome without a character-strengthening infusion of spiritual values as provided by caring mentors, therapists and groups. Otherwise, the patient may be sentenced to an unrewarding life with periodic fits of cruelty and self-destruction.

Spiritual Practices

Achieving spiritual awareness comes spontaneously to those who have highly sensitive spiritual receptors, particularly if they are put in challenging situations that open the channels between the egocentric self and the spiritual self. If, however, the spiritual receivers are in sleep mode, then they have to be turned on with spiritual practices such as meditation, yoga, visualization, prayer, chanting, and exercise routines, all of which, if done properly, can induce a state of focused, heightened awareness in those who may not come by it spontaneously. Not the least of these methods is practicing an art form that is expressive of one's inmost self.

There are many manuals that describe these techniques in detail.[45] What they all have in common is a procedure for focusing attention exclusively on simple actions or wished-for outcomes, such as the breathing process and wish-fulfilling visualizations, while discarding all distracting images, thoughts and feelings. With enough practice, the seeker has the opportunity to achieve an altered state of energized, heightened awareness outside of time and place. In this state, individuality recedes to give a glimpse of our common being and its connection to the "world soul," that is, to Spirit. I will leave it to the individual reader to find those approaches that best fit their individual personalities. Visualization of desired outcomes supplemented by vigorous exercise routines is all that is required for most of my patients, but others have found yoga, prayer, and martial arts, among other practices, uniquely conducive to achieving spiritual consciousness.

Conclusions

Spiritual therapy starts and ends with the aim of spiritual growth. We therapists encounter our patients as spiritual beings in need of understanding and activation. We diagnose their ailments from the medical, psychosocial, and spiritual frameworks, and we offer treatment that addresses these various dimensions as well as we can. To the extent that we succeed, the patients' will to health and faith is exponentially activated until they become creative moral agents that fight to repair their own souls and the spiritual fabric of the world, without suffering an overweening need for public recognition.

The root disease that stunts the growth of the tree of life, with its free, loving will, is severe biological anxiety, depressive, and cognitive disorder. The trunk infestation of this withered tree is psychological damage[46] deriving from early traumas that have caused dissociative splitting and from rearing practices that have fostered habits of passive inertia or spiteful defiance. The sparsely leafed, deformed limbs of this stunted tree represent spiritual emptiness or loss of morale, deriving from a lack of an inspiring belief system conveyed by caring individuals and social networks that strengthen the resolve to love, heal, and create structures of ultimate meaning. Activating the obstructed will ideally follows a sequence of good medicine, insightful relearning and integration, and transcendent awareness and guidance by spiritual values.

Chapter 5
THE DIVIDED WILL

Summary. Patients with the severe personality disorders, characterized by self-destructive acting out, have often suffered early physical and psychological trauma, the pain of which has been numbed by dissociative splitting. The splitting process leads to the formation of a divided self-will. In operational terms, this means that the healthy self's conscious plans for a successful love and work life are undermined by the machinations of an internal saboteur or abuser, which is responsible for serially reenacting the early traumatic experience that first led to the dissociative event. Because patients with a self-defeating internal saboteur or acting-out abuser typically have fundamental deficits in insight and will, they are usually unaware of the precise nature of their destructive behavior, and even if aware, they cannot curb it by utilizing their own unaided resources. Consequently, individual dynamic psychotherapy, which generally presupposes intact observing and executive ego (insight and will), might have to be supplemented by biological agents and a spiritually realized form of therapy, exemplified by a group network that provides auxiliary sources of observation and volition. Since the human psyche is an omniverse of complexity, it is unreasonable to assume that any symptom has a single cause that will respond to one technique. The spiritual therapy proposed here attempts to provide an integrated comprehensive framework of understanding and treatment that comes closer to taking the full measure of human suffering and its healing.

Disorders of the will come in several salient forms. Commonly seen in clinical practice are cases in which the will is paralyzed as a result of major depression or catatonic psychosis, typically characterized by a virtual shutdown of mental and physical activity. As in the example of Johanna (chapter 4), these individuals often do not have the energy or motivation to get out of bed or to initiate any action other than routine tasks. A second common type derives from war or sports injuries in which brain tissue has been destroyed, leaving victims without the functioning neural substrate either to conceive plans or to carry them out consistently and coherently. Then there are hyperactive, sometimes frenzied and disorganized forms of volition seen in ADHD and manic, hypomanic, and schizo-affective disorders. People with these instances of overactive will can be highly productive for periods of time but tend to suffer episodes of overreach and crash-and-burn that vitiate prior accomplishments, including their reputations for veracity and reliability.

Two significant forms of will impairment remain to be discussed: the blocked and the divided will. The blocked or obstructed will is best understood as an inhibition produced by psychological conflict. Needs and drives are blocked from achieving gratification typically by an inhibitory unconscious force in the personality such as a punitive, guilty superego. In Freud's theory the drive is often conflated with an oedipal wish: to do away with the father to have the mother all to oneself or to triumph over the mother to have the father. This activates a guilty conscience, which inhibits the drive's expression and thereby blocks the individual from achieving success.

In the larger, extra-therapy culture, blocked writers and composers are common subjects of biographies and memoirs. Novelist F. Scott Fitzgerald and composer Sergei Rachmaninov had significant periods of creative blockage, as did Rossini and Sibelius. We assume in these instances that the will to write or compose has been blocked by depression and psychological conflict, but since we do not typically have access to these artists' medical and psychiatric histories, our assumptions may be off the mark. Senile and alcoholic dementia, bipolar depression, and other clinical disorders are possible culprits in cases of creative paralysis.

This brings us back to the case of Doreen, discussed in the last chapter. As we recall, she could not write the dissertation for her PhD degree in sociology even though she had passed the preliminary exams and done the research supporting her thesis. By the time she finally withdrew from graduate school, she had spent almost eighteen years of futility, never able to sit down and do the writing. In our work together, we assumed that she suffered from a blocked will. She both loved and hated her father, and she hated the field of sociology, but she also wanted to redeem her father's ruined life and career as a sociologist by becoming one herself. Obviously there were enough conflicting motives here, including a guilty oedipal wish, to account for a blocked will. But the psychodynamic approach to resolving these conflicts, even bolstered by various medications, was totally ineffective. Toward the end of our work together, I realized that I had failed to deal adequately with a likely main cause of her failure. More than a blocked will, she had been manifesting the workings of a divided or split will. Not repressed conflict but split personality was the culprit. Moreover, she needed a dose of moral resolve to overcome her saboteur, a prescription I failed to write.

The importance of dissociation has proved to be a very contentious subject in the annals of psychiatry. It was the apparent cause of the rupture between the French psychiatrist Pierre Janet, the pioneer in the study of the dissociative mechanism, and Freud, who ultimately renounced his debt to Janet in understanding hysteria in favor of his own theory of repressed conflicts. Since Freud became the most influential modern authority in the field of therapy, Janet's contribution was a sideline issue to most clinicians trained in the first two-thirds of the twentieth century. Adding to the disfavor was the popular confusion as to the meaning of "split personality." For the longest time, lay people assumed that "split personality" referred to schizophrenic patients, not to those with acting-out personality disorders. For want of a stationary, well-defined target, the label was dispensed with in reputable training programs. To make matters worse, many psychiatrists and therapists of the late twentieth century became obsessed with the dissociative phenomena of multiple personality disorder (MPD) as the presumed last bastion of the pure psychogenic theory of psychiatric symptoms. The MPD diagnosis was overused to the point that therapists subtly began to influence patients to produce the florid symptoms of this overhyped disorder, to the mutual satisfaction of all concerned. Patients with the most numerous and bizarre "alter egos" became the stars of clinical conferences. The credibility of psychiatric diagnosis took a serious hit.

Split versus Shattered Will

More serious are cases of shattered wills, where the protective defense of dissociation has not been deployed effectively enough to ward off psychotic crumbling and flameout. We say of these individuals that their ego, self, or will has been broken in pieces, typically as a result of unbearable torture, abuse, isolation, personal losses, or maiming on the battlefield or playing field. Without expert care, they tend to remain too unstable and unfocused to make coherent plans or to exert the sustained resolve to realize them. At their untreated best, they become chaotic and rudderless, sometimes lapsing into catatonic-like states. If the whole armamentarium of spiritual therapy is used, victims of these traumas can sometimes be given enough purpose and faith, once a modicum of physical and mental integrity has been restored, to lead a life worth living. Service animals have sometimes proven effective in grounding these unfortunate individuals.

In categorizing these cases, the standard diagnosis of post-traumatic stress disorder (PTSD) focuses on the manifest symptoms of anxiety, hyperarousal, reliving or flashbacks, nightmares, and outbursts of rage. Less well recognized but a potentially more devastating consequence of trauma is the loss of spirit. One patient described this process vividly. After being president of his high school's student council and quarterback of its football team, he was rejected by a girlfriend, which led first to depression and then to hypomania and finally to what he described as "the feeling that my vitality was flowing right out of me." Now comparatively bland and unmotivated, he was cajoled and guided, mostly by his parents, into learning a trade and leading a life of routine order.

The Dissociated, Split Will

By successfully using the mechanism of dissociation, individuals can avoid shattering the will by splitting off the traumatized part and preserving a residual functioning self. Dissociation works like a circuit breaker that prevents the psychotic burnout of the self-will circuitry. But preserving a functioning conscious self comes at a high cost. The residual self is diminished in passion because dangerously strong feelings are exiled into the split-off part. More importantly, the dissociated part is typically enraged and bent on seeking revenge against the traumatizing agent, often judged to be the guilty residual self. Now the conscious residual self has to contend with a hateful subpersonality, which takes the form of an internal saboteur or often an external abuser. This saboteur or abuser serially reenacts the original traumatic incident and the vengeful retribution. It does this by looking out for or setting up situations that are reminiscent of the prototypical situation and then doing its damage, often in the most ingenious ways.

In chapter 2, I foreshadowed the workings of a split-off internal saboteur in discussing the case of Carl. The traumatic incident that set Carl's dissociative process in motion was his father's suicide just when his pubertal sexual and aggressive drives were kicking in. His split-off saboteur became enraged against him and exposed him to the possibility of injury, sickness, or death every time he tried to have a romantic relationship or to act assertively. Carl's weakened conscious self was an inviting target because he felt guiltily responsible for his father's death and therefore deserving of punishment. Fortunately, he retained a strong will to health, comprised of a "survival instinct" or "guiding spirit," that saved him from the catastrophic consequences of his numerous self-attacks. Auto accidents, bike accidents, episodes of gastrointestinal symptoms, attacks of scruples over mild attempts at self-assertion—these occurred so often in the early stages of treatment that they derailed most of his attempts to have an intimate relationship and later to protect himself from an abusive spouse.

Review of Common Types of Trauma

As indicated previously, children are very liable to suffer these catastrophic injuries to the self if a parent dies or is destroyed as a role model at crucial developmental phases, particularly if the event occurs in the context of the child's major stages of psychosexual and psychosocial development. This is also true in cases of traumatic physical or sexual abuse by parents, stepparents, siblings, and revered authority figures such as coaches and members of the clergy. Natural disasters and brutal warfare, characterized by overwhelming losses of security, physical integrity, the lives of loved ones, and homes and sources of livelihood, can similarly cause shattering or splitting of the self and will, adequately described in some cases by the diagnosis of PTSD. The dissociative by-products of overwhelming stress can also include a suicidal or homicidal partial self, which raises the chances of a deadly outcome. We have seen this all too often in soldiers returning from the Iraq and Afghanistan wars. Whether due to poor follow-up care or inadequate services and facilities in the war zones, the number of suicides or episodes of violence in this group is truly appalling.

One of my patients, a businessman, was physically and mentally abused often as an adolescent by his father, who had formerly seemed "normal" but who returned from the Korean War manifesting the post-traumatic effects of having been tortured by immersion in submerged cages, where water rodents bit off chunks of his flesh, similar to the graphic representations in the movie *The Deer Hunter*. With little provocation, he often struck my patient with a shovel or pierced his body with a pitchfork while calling him a "worthless piece of shit." Since no amount of medication can repair the broken will that results from such traumas, even though mood stabilizers and cognitive-enhancing antipsychotics[47] may give a boost, we are thrown back on the arduous work of freeing and strengthening a self-will that has been compromised by traumatic dissociation. In this case the consequences for my patient included lowered self-esteem and character strength and a heightened vulnerability to the workings of a self-defeating and proto-homicidal partial self. In addition to sabotaging some of his work projects, he became frighteningly abusive toward everyone with whom he became romantically involved. Now on his third try at marriage, with the help of treatment, he has managed to stay with his current wife for more than twenty years. Managing his psychic dissociation depended not only on recognizing its existence but also on following a program of training his will to anticipate and divert his internal saboteur's destructive acting out. The energy required to accomplish this feat had the unwanted effect of diminishing the romantic passion characteristic of his past disruptive love relationships, but this was a loss he was willing to accept in return for the gain in stability of his marriage. In a recent follow-up letter (May 2012), he wrote, "[We] are a couple and she continues to be the love of my life."

Dissociation and Personality Disorders: Lying or Unknowing

I want to go into more detail in showing how disorders of will are manifested in severe personality disorders, particularly those that exhibit dissociation and acting out. To begin with, we must emphasize again that dissociation is common and that its effects can be highly dangerous. This is because, as we have seen, splitting may give birth to a partial self—a subpersonality—that is capable of murder or suicide. We see this not only in everyday self-destructiveness represented by the cases we have discussed but also in horrific examples of homicide reported in the media, such as the case of Jeffrey McDonald, the Green Beret doctor who was found guilty of killing his pregnant wife and children some years back. He proclaimed his innocence with such earnestness that eminent forensic psychiatrists were convinced that he was telling the truth, that he was the victim of a miscarriage of justice. I am mindful of the possibility that new evidence may justify this position. But let us for the moment entertain the possibility that McDonald did commit the murders but genuinely believes that he did not. Once we admit the importance of dissociative splitting, intentional lying is not the only alternative to telling the truth. Rather than telling a simple lie, McDonald may no longer have any awareness of his actions because he dissociated the experience from consciousness and therefore believes his own story.

Joe McGinniss, in his book *Fatal Vision*, describes in gripping detail how he initially believed McDonald's account, only later to become convinced of his guilt by the accumulation of condemning evidence.[48] Since I have enormous respect for the forensic psychiatrists who think otherwise, I leave open the possibility that the case is merely suggestive evidence of my hypothesis but not entirely immune to reasonable doubt.

Once we recognize the possibility that a split-off part of the self might be capable of disowned actions, we begin to recognize the traces of a dissociated subpersonality in many accounts of fraudulent and destructive behavior—both in the clinical setting and as reported in the news media. I vividly recall the case of a Vietnam veteran who had machine-gunned his own squadron mates, a fact he stoutly denied. Recognizing that he was in dissociative denial, military psychiatrists at Walter Reed Hospital elected to strengthen rather than heal the split in his self and thereby avoid precipitating the psychosis that surely would have resulted from bringing the episode back into consciousness. Subsequently treating him in my home office—the referral source, his psychiatric-nurse wife, made no mention of his killing spree—turned out to be a harrowing experience and a good argument against treating all-comers in a home office. When his wife separated from him after making the referral, he held me responsible for her "betrayal" and went on a fist-shaking accusatory rant against me that became the stuff of subsequent nightmares. Getting him out of my office without getting hurt may have been my signal accomplishment in this case. Only after I described this episode to his wife did she come clean about his past history. She also took out a restraining order and alerted her local police to swing by her house with increased frequency.

A similar mechanism with a better outcome operated in the case of a man who found himself repeatedly and almost irresistibly veering into oncoming highway traffic, only with great effort pulling his car back into the right lane. Knowing from our therapy together that he had a split-off self-destructive partial self, manifested in other situations, was of significant assistance in helping him win the struggle against this enemy within.

Cases of actual or potential suicide and homicide are in fact not the most common forms of destructive acting out seen in private practice. I mention them to sound the alert to their existence and the dangers inherent in the will becoming divided. More common and relevant to our discussion are cases of split-off partial selves who, rather than commit murder or suicide, perpetrate various forms of mental and physical abuse and financial fraud. When the abuse is mainly self-directed, we call the subpersonality an internal saboteur. When it is other-directed, we say that the partial self is a tormentor or abuser of others. Note that all these terms involving abuse are morally laden judgments and therefore properly fit within a moral-spiritual framework. Try as we might to be pure empirical scientists, when we judge that patients are sabotaging or acting out abusively, we are morally convicting them—using words that imply they are behaving immorally, not just badly in the pragmatic sense of not getting what they or others want or need, but badly in the absolute sense of causing harm to themselves or others that is not deserved. No matter how much we protest to the contrary, we are not making value-free clinical judgments here.

This is particularly the case when we are confronted with the perpetrators of Ponzi schemes, some of whom think of their work as philanthropic. We do not hesitate to call them psychopaths, whether or not they know what they have done. As egregious as the recent Bernard Madoff scandal, although less costly to the victims, was the New Era Philanthropy scheme, the brainchild of John G. Bennett Jr., a self-avowed Christian businessman who bilked friends and their prestigious acquaintances, including both a former US Treasury secretary and the board chairman of the Philadelphia Orchestra, of over $350 million from 1989 to 1995, when the pyramid collapsed and he was forced to declare bankruptcy. All the while, this psychopathic "philanthropist" created an aura of great goodwill and moral rectitude. One of his intended targets told me, "He didn't sound right; something was fishy about his pitch, so I wasn't going to give him any of my money." Good moral sensitivity, I would say.

More about Splitting as Defense and Its Treatment

Let us remind ourselves that the initial act of splitting is designed not to do harm but rather to diminish the intolerable pain of feeling traumatized. That the product of splitting turns out to be destructive is an unintended consequence of the dissociative process. In an important sense, as the aforementioned case of "friendly fire" against squadron mates suggests, dissociation is a defense mechanism used to ward off development of psychosis, to avoid suffering personality disintegration. In the setting of severe, intolerable physical and emotional trauma, the individual splits in order not to shatter, with dissociation serving as a circuit breaker that avoids psychosis, typically at the cost of generating the symptoms of post-traumatic stress and acting-out partial selves. The traumatized self numbs its unbearable pain by splitting off the pain-bearing part from consciousness. This split-off part then develops a life of its own, typically as a hurt, enraged destroyer that gets triggered to come out—at best confined to nightmares and flashbacks, at worst exploding into destructive acting out—by situations that evoke memories of the original traumatic episodes. Then the whole process of reenactment begins.

Reenactment

To do justice to the fruitfulness of the conception, the theory of early dissociation and later reenactment needs to be fleshed out by clinical examples. Take the case of Howard, who pulled out of every relationship after a girlfriend's declaration of love. His childhood was characterized by severe emotional neglect by an alcoholic mother who, when not drunk, was incapacitated by an inflammatory bowel disorder. The first time he remembers going numb occurred when he was around five or six. His mother was holding him on her lap. He was gagging from the smell of alcohol on her breath, but when he tried to pull away, his mother reproached him tearfully: "Why can't you be more loving?" He felt an intolerable burning in his chest, and then he went numb. Soon thereafter, he stopped eating with the family, instead preparing his own meals and taking them to his room. As an adult, he interpreted any girlfriend's declaration of love as a depriving demand for him to be affectionate, throwing his saboteur into a cold rage, as if to say, "Where was your love and empathy when I really needed them and all you could do was make demands and smell bad? If you hadn't been so sick, I would have smashed your face."

As I discussed in *The Freedom of the Self*,[49] Howard partially overcame this pattern when he met Beth, formerly a mobster's girlfriend, who mixed her displays of affection with acts of rejection, such as always returning his presents or calling him disparaging names. The week before he became involved with Beth, he picked out from a crowd of 30,000 Phillies fans a rowdy flirtatious woman and asked her for a date. He canceled when he discovered that she, like his mother, suffered from alcoholism and inflammatory bowel disease. Based on this instance of synchronicity coupled with his persistent complaints of loneliness, I assumed that Howard was now ready for a serious relationship and therefore encouraged him to follow his inclination to pursue Beth. They managed to get married, have children, and stay together for eighteen years before the combined efforts of their resurgent saboteurs and the erosion of the scaffolding I had initially provided to bind the marital relationship together finally succeeded in tearing the fabric of their family bonds. For many of those years, they allowed me to splint their relationship by means of medication and individual, marital, and group therapy. But such interventions, with their attendant intrusiveness, are sustainable for only a finite length of time. They depend for their permanent success on the naturally strengthening bonds between the individuals themselves, which failed to solidify in this case.

Marriage as a Spiritual Phenomenon

Given the eventual breakup of Howard's marriage, was such intrusive splinting of the connection worth the effort? The answer depends in part on one's values, particularly spiritual values. I believe that if individuals want to get married and have a family but cannot sustain a relationship long and well enough to do so, then spiritually inclined therapists should pull out all stops to help them get the job done. Beyond declaring one's love for another and propagating the species by having offspring, the essential purpose of marriage is to achieve a sacred union—biologically, psychologically, and spiritually— with another soul and thereby open the way to achieving union with the timeless Self—that is, with Spirit as a whole. In the process, one transcends the limitations of the empirical ego and its earthly existence. Marriage in its fullest sense is not two people sealing a secular contract before a justice of the peace but rather is an exchange of vows in front of a symbolic community of loved ones—a spiritual group—that makes the union sacred. Instead of a contract, spiritually sanctioned marriage is a covenant, unbreakable except as the lesser of two evils: to save a life or a soul.

More about Multiple Personality Disorder

Note that such accounts of sabotage and abuse by subpersonalities are a far cry from the lurid accounts of multiple personality disorder that were so popular a few years back. After the publication of *The Three Faces of Eve* and the story of *Sybil*, the lay public and even many therapists tended to associate splitting with the coming out of completely new personalities who showed tendencies completely alien to the host character.[50] In such cases we encounter the prudish schoolteacher whose alter egos come out on weekends, leading her to wantonly pick up strangers in bars and steal from her colleagues at work, or the respectable family man who in the middle of the night silently escapes his sleeping wife to knock over all-night convenience stores and at other times is the first responder to neighborhood disasters.

Such cases are rarely seen in clinical practice. In fact, most multiple personalities are elaborated in the service of the interests of therapists who subtly coax patients into producing them. More common are not these fully developed alternative personalities but the fragmentary subpersonalities that we have been discussing. They have a much more limited set of objectives than true multiple personalities. Most often, they are rightly called internal saboteurs because they function like sleepers or moles: enemy agents who gum up our plans occasionally, not every day but from time to time. Sometimes becoming conscious and posing as our best selves, they soon demonstrate that they are alien, evil forces intent on sabotaging our ambitions. Internal saboteurs undermine the central self's conscious intentions. What is remarkable about them is that they have a will of their own, operating outside our awareness and control and bent on doing life-altering damage to us. Since this is not a popular idea, having nowhere near the currency of Freudian ideas about the workings of unconscious anger or libido, I digress here to give an expanded conception of unconscious volition, including some of its history.

The Freudian Lineage

Freud's spiritual predecessor, the German philosopher Schopenhauer (1788-1860), maintained that we ourselves are (unconsciously) bringing about what seems to be happening to us.[51] As the Schopenhauer-inspired novelist Thomas Mann put it, we are the secret playwrights and unwitting directors of our lives. In this sense, every personal history is actually self-written. The contents of our more-or-less objective biographies are, to a large extent, autobiographies. We are always secretly but willfully writing our own life story. No matter how much we feel we are the victims, we are actually the authors of our fate. Freud's contemporary, Pierre Janet, came up with a theory of dissociation that accounted for these unconscious enactments far more thoroughly than Freud's theory of repression, which applied mainly to feelings and conflicts rather than fully plotted actions. To our loss, Freud disparaged Janet's findings and put forward his more influential but less powerful fluid-dynamic model of instinctual repression, which held sway until the theory of dissociation regained its rightful place in contemporary personality theory. Freud also rejected the existence of spiritual or suprapersonal forces acting on the empirical field. As a result of this reductionism, many psychodynamic therapists have been left without the explanatory tools to account for extraordinary examples of either altruism or mass murder. Everything comes down to love versus hate as a result of good or bad mothering—with a slight nod to possible genetic influences. This trivialization of human motivation is being rectified as the reality of spiritual experience steadily regains its rightful place in contemporary personality theory and practice, along with a greater appreciation of neurochemical and neurophysiological variations in behavioral causation.

Patterns of Self-Defeat

The kernel of truth to be found in the theory that we are bringing about what happens to us should not blind us to its limitations. One-of-a-kind events often fall outside this purview. For instance, a blind, physically maimed woman worked out at my health club. She had suffered a brain injury from a flower pot dropped accidentally from an upper story. It would be both cruel and fruitless to suggest that she had somehow, through her unconscious will or in retribution for past misdeeds, brought this upon herself. How can it be construed as self-destructive to walk on a city sidewalk in a good neighborhood? In everyday life, we accomplish very little by giving serious consideration to the possibility that our participation in a common will, bent on retribution for past sins, is somehow at work to produce these apparently senseless tragedies.

Instead, I suggest that this hypothesis is best applied to repetitive patterns of behavior, to people's characteristic successes and failures. In these cases, we are enjoined by Schopenhauer—and more relevantly, by Freud's clinical application—to examine what part the individual's unconscious will may have played in bringing about destructively patterned events. Even within its restricted application, the notion remains so disturbing as to demand further clarification.

The idea that we create our own destiny may seem less problematic when good things keep coming our way. We tend to say that we are "lucky" or the beneficiaries of serendipity. It is not too much of a stretch to think that our own will, or at least our personal merits, might have something to do with it. Perhaps the Calvinist notion applies: that our wealth and good fortune are signs of divine favor. Yet since we have been taught from childhood not to entertain such self-serving thoughts, we tend to slide over the origins of good fortune, feeling little need to inquire into its causes. We just shake our heads in wonderment and hope the good times keep rolling.

But we cannot avoid looking for an explanation when bad things continually hound us. Do we somehow deserve such misfortune, or are we the victims of a cruel, impersonal fate? Some people really may be unlucky. They are born with a crippling congenital defect, low intelligence, bad looks, or severe mental illness, and then life dumps one affliction after another on their heads. Again, we must look to theology and metaphysics, as well as statistics, for explanations of such manifest unfairness; it serves no therapeutic purpose to compound the injustice by casting blame on the victim. Of course, praise should be given in abundance when someone rises above adversity to develop strong character and lead a productive life.

We first become suspicious that we might be causing our own troubles when we see ourselves responding destructively to success. We all know people whose every accomplishment is followed by an equal or greater failure. For example, a business executive has started three highly successful chains of clothing stores, earning millions of dollars each time. But in each case, he has overexpanded and driven the business into bankruptcy. Time after time, a large success is followed by a crash. Why does this keep happening? His associates described frequent mood swings, at their worst rendering him incapable of acting rationally. To attribute the pattern entirely to a bipolar mood disorder is an insufficient explanation. There are after all many consistently successful business executives and professionals with bipolar disorders who know better than to let their moods dictate their actions; at the very least they surround themselves with trusted handlers to whom they listen. The fact remains that others cannot accept that they are liable, if left uncurbed, to serially author destructive scenarios.

My own experience in treating these crash repeaters is that coming to such awareness in a way that stops the repetition is so painful that the insight is strongly resisted. Characteristic mood swings from manic grandiosity to depressive self-loathing erect great barriers to self-awareness. Moreover, some who manage to grasp the pattern intellectually are often unable to change the behavioral outcome. One patient went through three bankruptcies on my watch. He could never give warning when he was about to make a foolish investment. Afterward, he would chastise himself for being pathetic. Seeing that we are the cause of our own losses but being unable to stop losing is just one more self-defeat added to a résumé, and perhaps the most painful one of all.

And the barrier to understanding is even greater when the "unlucky" patterning is less obviously an undoing of prior successes. For example, Howard, unable to sustain a relationship, as discussed earlier,[52] had no lasting success to be offset by a subsequent failure. Rather, Howard kept encountering a barrier to realizing his most cherished conscious goal of getting married and having a family. In these common patterns, patients initially claim that they have so far failed to find the right partner, not that they themselves might be arranging the failure.

Similarly, after a series of job fiascos, patents may complain about bureaucratic bungling and office politics, which may in fact be factors, but they cannot initially admit the further possibility that they are laying themselves open to getting fired by repeated misbehaviors, that they may be bringing about what seems to be happening to them. The blow to self-esteem of recognizing our own bungling is typically too painful to admit. And it's a hard sell for the therapist to get the message across. Yet this is a necessary step in stopping the pattern. The essential steps that must be taken to overcome the workings of internal saboteurs or abusers are outlined in what follows.

The Four Steps

1. *Identify the acting-out pattern.* Most commonly, this involves coming to recognize how we alienate our superiors or friends or how we get ourselves thrown out of jobs or schools, all by characteristic missteps that would ordinarily be within our abilities to avoid. The worst cases, as illustrated by Carl and Howard's stories, involve repeated accidents or otherwise blowing up love relationships that we desperately want and need. There is no denying the fact that we cannot ordinarily identify these patterns of failure without outside help. No matter how "well analyzed" we presume to be, our capacities for making self-serving rationalizations get in the way of seeing what we are doing. And it is potentially shattering to look unflinchingly into the mirrors of our actions because traumatic past experiences might be evoked, as we will soon discuss. Therefore, we need helpers who make it possible for us to see and bear the pain of seeing. For more than a century now, such helpers have come

from the ranks of professional therapists, which I believe to be altogether a good thing, since friends and loved ones are rarely objective enough (or have permission) to do the job. Among professional therapists I believe that those with a spiritual orientation have the best chance of offering this insight in a way that avoids permanent damage to the true self and, in particular, to its channels to Spirit. Such therapists frame these repeated patterns of defeat not as failures but as misconceived plans that prepare us for correcting them and putting us on the path to a better life. By doing so the therapists are able to offer hope of overcoming bad behaviors without skirting the issue of those behaviors' being bad and destructive. Sometimes, as in Carl's case, a member of the clergy may offer a seemingly magical absolution.

2. *Stop the acting out by persuasion, limit-setting, and response-prevention.* Take the case of Guillermo. Every time he got near to patching up his relationship with Isabel, he would start an easily discovered extramarital affair. After getting him to acknowledge the pattern, I gave him the support and the picture of dire consequences needed to persuade him to desist from going through with the impending infidelity. I called on his group members to mount a round-the-clock preventive watch. As a consequence of the thwarting of his acting out, he developed a severe depressive episode with signs of impending psychotic decompensation. The acting-out pattern was traced to the trauma of an early family disruption caused by his parents' divorce. Infidelities became an acting-out method of avoiding the crushing pain of reexperiencing this traumatic injury to the self, stimulated by the possibility of a realized close relationship with its attendant increased risk of loss. Stopping the acting out put him in touch with the unbearable pain that had caused the initial split in the self. Splitting and its acting-out expression functioned as a circuit breaker that protected him from shattering. Splitting is one of the two most powerful defenses against the psychotic shattering of the self, the other being obsessive-compulsive ritualizing.

3. *Assuage the underlying core distress, typically an intolerable agitated or enraged psychotic depression.* The pain of impending breakdown is what is exposed when the acting-out expression of the defensive split is curbed. Doris, a physician, could never become enamored of an appropriate partner because to do so would put her in touch with the intolerable pain of her mother's perceived rejection for passionately loving her father in her oedipal and early adolescent stages. Instead she would turn cold and contemptuous of her partners, especially after having agreed to marry them. Under my supposedly watchful eye, she did this on two successive occasions. When her group and I

made attempts to prevent her from going through with her second marriage to Sam, an uneducated hospital orderly with addictive tendencies, she became agitated and inconsolable, speaking in near-delusional terms of destroying his life. In addition to prescribing additional medication and intensive group support, we had no choice but to watch her go through with the wedding, a marriage that ended in divorce only two years later. In other cases, appropriate medication, crisis intervention, increasing frequency of sessions, and group support will sometimes stem the tide of these headlong jumps into the abyss. As with stopping any addictive or irresistible impulse, calling upon the greater will of the unified Self is often essential to success. This is why a community of the faithful offering support is correlated so highly with abstinence from these patterns of destructive behavior. Unfortunately this was not the case with Doris.

4. *Learn healthier patterns of resolving conflicts and achieving more beneficial results.* There is no more painful conflict than being pulled in different directions by a conscious self on the one hand and a subpersonality with a different agenda on the other. Once we are made conscious that part of us wants to cheat, steal, lie, or betray, and the healthy part of us wants to honor our commitments and observe the other tenets of the moral code, we are desperate to find the means to resist the temptation to act out. Aware that he had a preternatural sex drive, a renowned minister charged his assistants with making certain that he was never left alone with a female admirer. Instead he used his seductive spirit to convert both men and women to religious faith and to submit his instinctual life to a higher power of control. To subdue his tendency for outbursts of physical aggression, a former football player learned a martial art and taught it to young men and women who needed to curb similarly aggressive tendencies. Needless to say, these healthy resolutions of enactments born of conflict require not only some awareness of impending trouble but also the placement of barriers to stop the train before it rushes out of the station.

Awareness alone may come too late to do any good. Prizefighter Sugar Ray Robinson said that in his prime he was aware only of seeing his opponents hit the canvas. In his later slowed-down days, he saw openings in his opponent's defenses and made decisions to swing. By that time it was he himself who hit the canvas. Perhaps the appropriate barrier here was not better awareness but earlier retirement.

Treatment Barriers

The therapeutic pessimism that hovers over the treatment of severe personality disorders derives from the fact that these steps, particularly the first three, are strongly resisted by most patients and, to some extent, the field of therapy itself. Let me elaborate.

Identifying the pattern is often thwarted by patients' inability to cooperate in the discovery. By definition they do not know *that* or *how* they are acting out, only that they keep getting into trouble. They often cannot give an accurate report of what they are doing to cause these troubles. As I will discuss shortly, patients' blind spots about their behavior, which makes them poor historians, typically cannot be overcome without introducing an outside observer into the acting-out social field.

Stopping the identified acting-out pattern is strongly resisted by patients because indulging it brings relief from underlying anxiety and depression, and renouncing it leads to the intolerable foreshadowing of tearing the fabric of the self. For example, Phyllis knows that having contact with her abusive ex-husband, who treats her much like her own parents have always treated her, will shred her self-esteem and impede her chances of finding a better partner. But my strongly worded advice to avoid him and also to limit contact with her parents long enough to gain some emotional independence is followed for only three or four weeks before she acquiesces to meet with her ex and to be told once again that her "butt is too fat" or that her "hair is a mess." The resulting hurt feelings do not fire up strong enough willpower for her to rise above the initial sense of devastating loss that follows and to stop these encounters and recognize that they are reenactments of early parental abuse. But only by such acts of will can there be any healing of the deep wounds to the self that these self-destructive actions both protect and manifest. The frequently made comparison of these compulsive patterns to addictive behavior is especially apt. The craving for an addictive substance is rarely stronger than a yen for these masochistic experiences. Despite all the support I could muster, Phyllis chose to stop treatment rather than endure the distress of resisting her behavior pattern. She declined the offer to join one of my groups or to seek the spiritual support of a twelve-step program devoted to destructive sexual addictions.

Assuaging the underlying hurt exposed by stopping the acting-out pattern is problematic because the suffering is often of such traumatic intensity that relief must be immediately forthcoming. Otherwise, the patient is in imminent danger of psychotic decompensation, and therefore there is a risk he or she will bolt from therapy altogether to avoid the intolerable pain of a psychic shattering. Averting these disasters often necessitates emergency meetings, late-night phone sessions, and immediate doses of antianxiety and antipsychotic medications, as well as other medical and psychosocial interventions. Not the least of these interventions may be a group meditation in which both the pain and its solace are enjoined in the united Self. We therapists are often caught off-guard by the dangerousness of the situation and are unprepared to intervene with sufficient speed and force. Not only must medication and psychological understanding be urgently and expertly provided, but huge doses of emotional support also must be dispensed to walk the patient through the process successfully. To provide spiritual healing, calling together the patient's social network, sometimes including the clergy, on an emergency basis is often vital to repairing the integrity of the self.

The fourth step, developing a new repertoire of behaviors, is a less acute, longer-range goal. Someone such as Phyllis, for example, would have to force herself to spend time with men who do not abuse her and who therefore might not trigger her masochistic pleasure. If she can be supported in not giving in to her desire to run from these "boring" dates, she might in time come to appreciate less harmful if initially less stimulating partners.

Because of the difficulty in accomplishing these steps, patients and therapists understandably become discouraged and lose hope of reversing the destructive patterns. But at a time when the mental health professions have a larger arsenal of effective techniques than ever before, the key to greater success in treating severe personality disorders is for therapists to master a sound theoretical understanding of their etiology and an effective program of interventions, the carrying out of which requires a high quotient of pain tolerance, trust, and cooperation on the part of patients and an openness by all concerned to spiritual factors in sickness and healing.

Further Case Examples

Jack, in his late forties, had a series of relationships with women, all of whom canceled dates at the last minute or refused to have sex or see him anymore, rejections that always caught him by surprise. The prototype of this pattern occurred when he was about eight. His mother was hospitalized for a paranoid psychosis after giving birth to a child with Down syndrome.

Previously very loving toward Jack, or so he claims, she now was relentlessly critical, calling him selfish and the cause of his sister's birth defect. His adult love life became a reenactment of this rejection. To start with, he became involved only with women who demonstrated a tendency to reject, and then he would provoke them with inconsiderate behavior, suffering inconsolable rage and hurt over being accused or abandoned. When asked why he picked such rejecting partners, he claimed to be bored by women who were uncritically adoring. He lost interest in them after a few dates, often dismissing them rudely. This reminds us that reenactors are not confined to playing the victim in a reenactment; they can also play the perpetrator. Reenactments are replays of a whole situation, not just a single role in it.

Mary picked her boyfriends from those who expressed disinterest in ever getting married. Some of them changed their minds, but when they proposed, she would start a war of accusations or develop a severe psychosomatic condition, such as unrelenting neck pain, that required a great deal of doctoring. In the interest of health, she is now "permanently engaged" to Bruce. Every time they have talked about a wedding date, Mary has done her usual thing, or Bruce has had an accident himself. Until everyone agreed on a "terminal" engagement, one or both of them might come to my office in leg casts or neck braces. One new patient who passed them in my waiting room asked if my subspecialty was orthopedics.

Mary also tended to get fired at work after a promising start. At her most recent job, she was promoted and given a large bonus. The very next day, she accidentally deleted the results of her last several months' work. Although a computer expert was able to retrieve the data from her hard drive, Mary was shaken enough to make an emergency appointment. After the September 11, 2001, terrorist attack, she abruptly walked off the job because of her fear of a subsequent attack and refused to contact her boss, who sent word that he was willing to take her back. Although she found the notion of an internal saboteur working behind the scenes to create these self-defeats very illuminating and sparing of self-esteem, the dissociative events that initiated this pattern of presumed reenactment were never recovered. Nevertheless, she was ultimately able, by repeated acts of will, to curb enough of her saboteur's destructive behavior to keep her fiancé and subsequently to find and maintain a suitable job. I recently heard through the grapevine of former patients that Mary and Bruce finally got married after they both retired and terminated treatment!

In sum, what we are usually presented with in these cases is individuals with a divided or broken will, who manifest their disability by characteristic patterns of self-defeating behavior. As we have seen, they have blind spots about the nature of their behavior because it is split off from awareness. Trying to bring it into awareness resurrects the traumatic pain underlying the original splitting process. Because of these phenomena, repairing a broken will requires special treatment arrangements. Before the necessity of crisis intervention, we may have to set up certain evocative conditions that throw light on patients' blind spots while at the same time guarding against triggering pain that would prove too damaging without immediate caring support and treatment.

The Conditions of Treating Dissociative Reenactment

Introducing Observers

As with repression, dissociation renders individuals unaware of the motives, patterns, and impacts of their behavior. They have blind spots. For instance, Al, a very methodical attorney, had over 130 consecutive dates after he divorced (see chapter 10), but only two women agreed to go out with him a second time. He accepted the usual explanations—not really being ready to date, the reappearance of an old flame, new travel or work schedule—but his group members knew that his negative demeanor must be playing a part. Since he was, despite his negativity, a likable person, there had to be more to it. How to find out? Although therapists trained in the psychodynamic tradition expect the off-putting behavior to manifest in the therapeutic relationship—if not in individual therapy, certainly in the more evocative format of the therapeutic group—we are often unable to detect the pattern when the saboteur, like all good spies, has "deep penetration" and special chameleon-like skills, honed over the years, to escape detection.

The method I have developed to flush out the saboteur is to insert an observer into the patient's outside life, who has the patient's permission to report to his or her group. I suggested that Al escort Sarah, a fellow group member and former professional singer, to the amateur jazz club at which she often performed. Since he did not seem romantically interested in her, Sarah asked an attractive single friend to join them. Al proceeded to interrogate her in a nasty, smart-alecky way: "Are you a supervisor, or do you do real work? How smart are you? Why have you stayed so long in a dump like Philly?" He also corrected her for calling him a lawyer instead of an attorney. While committing these boorish acts, he failed to discover that she was a hiker and mountain climber, interests that he shared, and that she had just returned from climbing Kilimanjaro. After the encounter, the friend told Sarah that Al was "the most unpleasant man [she had] ever met." Al was shocked and deeply pained to learn that he had done these things and made this kind of impression, that the questions he had asked were taken seriously and found offensive. He reluctantly agreed to take an antidepressant for a brief period to get him through the pain of exposing the depressive wound instigating his behavior. After this breakthrough—this exposure of his saboteur's mischief—he was able to see that hostile interrogation or talk of the prestige of his Ivy League law education was not the best way to endear himself. But this was the kind of dining room conversation he had grown up with.

From Al's early years, his father had interrogated and argued with him constantly, often invoking parental authority when his facts were weak. These debates prepared Al for the practice of law but not a love life. And similar to Jack's case, Al's mother fell into a severe depression when he was a child. Previously the apple of his mother's eye, he was now shunted aside as his mother poorly coped with the loss of her own mother. He grew increasingly desperate and awkward in trying to recapture her attention, to no avail. As a compensation for his loss, he yearned to have a steady girlfriend as early as third grade, but he made all the wrong moves, like making hostile instead of friendly remarks. The response he provoked then was exactly the same kind of rejection he generated with his recent encounter at the jazz club and presumably on the numerous failed dates. With the benefit of insight, he described a sequence of feeling estranged from his date and falling back on trying to recapture the only kind of connection he knew, the argumentative one he had with his father. His former wife, also a litigious attorney, had been agreeable to this kind of relationship initially but had grown increasingly dissatisfied as her deeper needs went unmet. Soon after his saboteur's cover was blown, and he saw the pattern of his reliving, Al's dating history changed dramatically, and he became involved for the first time with an affectionate woman.

Similarly, Larry couldn't get a job even though he had a prestigious MBA and high-level financial skills. He was out of work almost two years before it occurred to me to send an observer on his job interviews. The watcher was a CPA who often helped my patients with their taxes and money problems. He discovered that Larry appeared very "shifty" in these interviews because he kept nervously scanning everyone's face, and he over-answered questions by going into needless detail, as if he were guilty of some offense that required special pleading. It was not difficult to locate the origins of this self-defeating behavior in his reaction to his parents' nasty divorce when he was seven, but more importantly, he was then able to rein in these tendencies enough to get an excellent job on the very next try.

The idea of introducing a watcher into the patient's outside life falls outside the bounds of traditional therapy. Not only are conventional therapists warned against socializing with individual patients, but patients also are not to socialize with each other or with appointed professionals outside the individual or group arrangement. The logic of this position would require us also to forbid family members from socializing outside the family or marital therapy sessions. Instead of always feeling bound by these rules, which are anachronistic in an age of social and milieu therapies anyway, let us recognize that there are dangers to extending therapy outside the walls of a clinic or private office, but that we just might have to accept the attendant risks if we intend to treat severe personality disorders effectively, given the personality flaws and saboteurs associated with these conditions.

Setting Limits

The acting out of internal saboteurs is not only self-defeating but also typically harmful to others. At the very least, victims of the patient suffer unearned rejection and exploitation and sometimes severe financial and emotional damage. The responsible therapist knows that such behavior must be stopped, first because it is the right thing to do, but also because the patient otherwise has no chance of getting well. "Setting limits" is the term we use for this kind of therapeutic intervention: the active curtailment of any destructive, symptomatic behavior but especially those reenacted behaviors that are self-defeating and harmful to others. The techniques of limit-setting, the subject of my first publication,[53] are worth reviewing because they are taught reluctantly or not at all in most therapy training programs. Explicitly utilizing such methods seems to go against the grain of a form of treatment and a type of society that pay lip service to being nondirective and nonjudgmental. The inadvisability of blindly pursuing such ideals becomes apparent every time an individual or a social entity goes completely out of control and becomes persecutory or murderous. Then the task is to reassert control with the least damage to the individual's or group's sense of worth and future capacity for self-governance.

So with apologies to the ghost of Carl Rogers, the promoter of nondirective therapy,[54] I maintain that destructive behavior must be curtailed if patients are to get better. And by destructiveness, I mean not only determinedly harmful actions but also the destructive fallout from depressive tactics, such as playing the martyr, and the chaotic behaviors of borderline and psychotic conditions. Yet since therapy is by definition a voluntary process occurring in a free society, this curtailment must be accomplished by persuasion rather than coercion. Persuasion is accomplished by a judicious combination of education and social pressure, which patients are always free to reject unless they are certifiably dangerous. As always, the specific mechanisms of setting limits are information, personal sanctions, medication, and structured activity.

Information. The gentlest form of limit-setting is to explain to patients the self-destructive consequences of their behavior, once the offending pattern has been identified and acknowledged. For some this simple insight into a previously obscure reality is surprisingly effective. They get it right away and make corrections. The appeal to reason is always the first option in dealing with free men and women whose autonomous decision making is held sacred. Unfortunately, it is not always so easy. Some require repeated demonstrations of the untoward effects of their saboteur's actions before they can activate the healthy will to rein it in. It may take a heart attack, a stroke, a DUI conviction—being hit by a two-by-four, as it were—to get their attention. If these demonstrations fail to limit the unhealthy behavior, then progressive penalties or sanctions may have to be imposed, the most powerful of which is the loss of cherished relationships, not only those losses naturally imposed by fed-up spouses and colleagues but also the relationship with the therapist and group members, who may have to make an offer the patient is loath to refuse. Needless to say, the therapist should never use such intimidating tactics unless there is no other way to avoid irreparable human tragedy.

Sanctions. Even though patients are not held responsible for their saboteurs' past actions, they are induced to take responsibility for their future misdeeds. So penalties legitimately come into play if this responsibility is shirked. In the realm of persuasion, a penalty is in the eye of the beholder; that is, it has to involve the prospect of the patient losing something that he or she values. This begins with an expression of the therapist's disapproval, which threatens the loss of his or her esteem if the offending behavior is not stopped. To repeat, the ultimate penalty is losing a love relationship. In the case of the therapeutic relationship, the threat may have to be made real if the circumstances are dire enough: "If you don't stop doing this, there is little point in our continuing to work together." As we shall discuss later, the threat may involve taking patients out of a highly valued therapeutic group without necessarily stopping individual therapy. In other situations making patients aware that their misbehavior is seriously endangering the continuing relationship with or even the welfare of a marital partner, child, parent, or friend often prods them to try harder to stop the bad pattern.

Not just close relationships but also health and livelihood may be endangered, and making this perfectly clear is often a powerful inducement to getting patients to bring their saboteurs under control. Making these threatened losses real eventualities—that is, presenting them to the patient's reason and imagination in a compelling way—is one of the crucial skills of the activist therapist, overlapping with the ability to cajole and prod the individual to walk a path that is radically different from those previously trod in order to have a better life. Sometimes this is not possible without use of medications to improve the biological substrate of disorder. As always, for the patient to swallow these bitter pills, spiritual attunement with a support system may be a necessary inducement.

Medications. As we have discussed before, symptoms of mood and thought disorders may impair the patient's will to take effective action, and this is particularly true when the required action is to oppose the workings of an internal saboteur or abuser. Blowing the saboteur's cover and laying bare the underlying traumatic wound to the self is a psychiatric emergency often requiring emergency antipsychotic maneuvers because of the emergence of intolerable pain that threatens disintegration of the personality. In the presence of depressive, disorganized, and destructive behavior, antidepressants, mood stabilizers, antipsychotics, and anxiolytics are prescribed to tilt the balance away from blind, maladaptive reflex to free, constructive choice. Needless to say, these medications should always be given with liberal amounts of spiritual support and heartfelt empathy. For the will to be activated in the fullest sense, medications must also be supplemented by an individually tailored program of organized striving.

Structured activity. For destructive behavior to be curbed, the will not only must be freed from the paralyzing effects of mood, thought, and dissociative disorders, but it also must be anchored in a matrix of productive rituals. These must be tailored to the individual's specialized needs and temperament. For some, the observances of organized religion may fill the bill. For others, spiritual practices including chanting, prayer, meditation, visualization, yoga, and martial arts are better fits. Note that all of these practices lie deep within the spiritual core of the great religions or nontheological philosophies of life such as Buddhism. What I have found to be basic in all physically able patients is an exercise program that is at base physically gymnastic but that can be done in the spirit of transcending the physical to become spiritually gymnastic—that is, a ritual that can open a door to a higher, creative vision. On a daily or several-times-weekly schedule, patients are urged to stake their life on fulfilling a prescribed program of mind-focusing exercise. Sit-ups, push-ups, and work on exercise machines, along with swimming, biking, rowing, jogging, and other aerobic activities, can all be structured into the patient's day to promote the desired benefits. To put it in the simplest terms, the discipline of mental and physical gymnastics strengthens both the body and the will, the conditioning of which no person who expects to rise above the symptoms of psychiatric disorders can afford to neglect. These activities are especially needed to overcome the potential for passive, magical thinking that taking potent psychoactive medications can engender. Active concentration on one point of consciousness during these exercise programs is essential.

Combining Individual and Group Therapy

Implicit in much of the foregoing discussion is that traditional individual therapy has proven to be an inadequate, incomplete approach to treating severe personality disorders. This is because the individual's powers of insight and will have been compromised by the presence of mood and thought disorders and split-off internal saboteurs. But insight and will—observing and executive ego in psychodynamic parlance—are preconditions of a therapy of psychological and spiritual growth. To put them in place, biological agents often have to be added to individual therapy to combat the medical components of disturbances in mood and thinking. And the individual format has to be supplemented by group methods, including family, marital, and milieu approaches, to invoke the larger, aggregate will of the spiritual self to overcome the weakening effects of dissociative splitting on the individual will. Only with the help of the group will can volitionally challenged individuals blow the cover of their saboteurs and then corral them and get them to work *for*, instead of *against*, the healthy, conscious self and—even more importantly— *for* the spiritual self. How does group therapy strengthen the individual will to achieve these goals?

Providing a source of outside observers. One way, already mentioned, is that the therapeutic group serves as a primary source of outside observers. Only because Al escorted Sarah to her singing gig and was introduced to her friend were we able to see Al's saboteur come out and block his chances for a successful relationship. In short, Sarah, a fellow group member, "outed" his saboteur. Although someone outside the therapy milieu might be able to perform this role, such as the accountant I sent along to monitor Larry's job interviews, this is difficult to arrange and much less likely to turn up someone with the requisite interests and observational skills. The observer introduced from the group may also play a crucial role in making the correct primary diagnosis. For example, before Beth and Howard developed a romantic relationship, Howard was reclusive, and Beth, a fellow group member, volunteered to take him to a party and introduce him to one of her girlfriends. Howard reported back that Beth had a few drinks, became wildly manic, took off some of her clothes, and did a lewd dance on a tabletop in the restaurant. Prior to that time, I had been treating Beth as an uncomplicated case of depression. Without Howard's information, I had little chance of bringing her destructive, manic behavior under control because she could not, or would not, report it, and I had not detected it in our private therapy sessions.

Evoking "holographic" patterns. Of course, if patients manifest their self-destructive behavior within the individual or group therapy relationships, there is no need to introduce outside observers to detect it, just as there might be no need to supplement individual therapy with group therapy. Self-centeredness, insensitivity, and deficits in reciprocity often become readily apparent in individual therapy, although they may become more obvious in the group setting. And certainly with no need for help from a group's observational skills it becomes readily apparent in individual work that some patients are overt about sabotaging their relationships—for example, by repeatedly missing or being late for appointments or by failing to pay bills or keep promises and lying about the reasons. For such gross lapses in responsibility, the possibility of doing any kind of therapy, individual, group, or biological, is thrown into doubt.

Nevertheless, the group format is ideally suited to evoking often subtle, personally meaningful destructive patterns, some of which I have called "holograms" in *The Freedom of the Self.* By a behavioral hologram, I mean a small piece of behavior that reveals the basic thrust of the individual's whole personality: its fundamental aims and values and its core pathology. In this sense, telling a racist or sexist joke in mixed company is a hologram of the teller's overall insensitivity, bad taste, chauvinism, or racial prejudice.

More to the point, after Al's love-destroying saboteur was revealed and limits were set on it, he fell in love with June, who was interested in marrying him. But instead of sharing his good fortune with the group, he began to report regularly on all the disasters that befell June, her family, and all his other relationships: for example, he relished telling that June's mother had a detached retina, that he had spent the night in the emergency room with the family, that his ninety-year-old father had become bland and confused after his heart operation, that a friend had died and left his estate in a mess, and on and on. Group members became increasingly put off by this recital of ruin that made him sound like an off-duty mortician. But this was a hologram of how Al always turned impending happiness into farcical tragedy, a pattern that he had inherited from his depressed mother in childhood. It was how his own characterological depression was operationalized: he squeezed the life out of all good happenings by concentrating on the dirtballs under the bed. But as a hologram it also pointed to the dark side of Spirit, where the lowest common denominator of group awareness aggregates to form the negative will of destructiveness. Warned that he was about to do with June what he had done with his last marriage, he began to change his patterns and become more adventurous and spontaneous about their time together. With encouragement from his group, he even abandoned his rigid timetable about when they might get engaged. The couple began to feel some enchantment in their travels and in the friends they made.

One of the reasons the group is such a potent evoker of destructive holograms is that it symbolically recreates the early family setting where such holograms typically originate. Repeatedly I have seen patients manifest their core pathology, which permeates everything they do, soon after entering a group. In the group, I stand for the father or mother of the family of origin, and fellow patients may stand for parents, siblings, housekeepers, and other members of the early social milieu. And in this symbolically realized family setting, new patients manifest the depressive, mistrustful, rebellious, and responsibility-shirking patterns they first developed to deal with their real families. Very few individual therapists have the stimulus value to evoke such a wide range of attitudes and behaviors in need of remediation.

Serving as sources of support. Confronting an internal saboteur is extremely painful. As we have mentioned, the splitting process leading to saboteur formation is an attempt to reduce intolerable, potentially shattering psychic pain. Exposing the split by thwarting and thereby "outing" the saboteur re-evokes this original pain, which cannot be tolerated without large doses of spiritual support and oftentimes medication. Group members who have reined in their own saboteurs and know how devastating the resulting pain can be are the most potent, effective sources of this support. Not only does the original pain of discovery require their sympathy and assuagement, but so do the changes that must be made to heal the split or at least to lessen its destructive impact. This sometimes involves emotionally distancing from hurtful parents or siblings, dissolving soul-destroying bad marriages, seeing less of previously close but now less congenial friends, and making career changes, all because these various relationships are elicitors of their saboteur's acting out and serve to strengthen the saboteur's influence on the person's life. The changes involved cannot always be accomplished unless the support of the individual therapist is supplemented by the much greater mass of group support. In dire circumstances, the course of action taken in the following case may have to be entertained, a truly horrible possibility that can be realized only with strong outside encouragement and binding of guilt by the spiritual group.

Marlene's mother could only be described as an evil person. She beat her children; made them do their own laundry at an early age; frequently threatened to abandon them and, as they got older, on several occasions called in an attorney to change her will in their presence; used imaginary ills to tyrannize them; and constantly humiliated their gentle father, destroying him as a role model. In order to break free of her mother's influence and allow herself to have a non-evil love life and spiritual life, Marlene decided to cut herself off completely from her mother, a step that was almost impossible to sustain when her mother was diagnosed with a terminal illness. She was devastated to listen to her mother's pleading voice mail messages as she lay dying. Marlene made certain that her sister and brother attended to her mother's basic needs during this period. Getting Marlene through it all required the full arsenal of therapeutic methods but most importantly the support of her group members, who sympathized with her pain and helped her justify an admittedly ruthless but necessary course of action. In effect, the group gave her absolution, not in a religious sense but in the sense of providing the level of justification and forgiveness that only a large, spiritually encompassing group will can provide.

Even so, Marlene was plagued by overwhelming guilt and often took to bed for days at a time. But she realized that in undoing her mother's influence in the only way she had not yet tried, she was fighting for the very existence of her soul. She was supported in her growing conviction that cutting herself off from her mother was the lesser of two evils. Even though it was a profound act of disloyalty and a violation of one of the most sacred moral commandments, it had the effect of strengthening her character and integrity. After a period of guilty bereavement, she began to enjoy a healthier and more fulfilling life.

Opening up to an enlarged, spiritual will. The group does more than give support. It provides an arena in which previously covert pathology is manifested, in which corrective feedback is offered, and in which issues brought up in individual sessions can be worked through. But more important than all these is its capacity to strengthen the broken, divided will, characteristic of patients with acting-out personality disorders. In the realm of addictive disorder, where the will is powerless to resist alcohol, overeating, narcotics, gambling, and promiscuous sex, the twelve-step programs have taught us how the group will overrides the destructive indulgences of the individual will. The recovery rate from addictive disorders is distressingly low at best and almost nonexistent without drawing on the will and spirit of an assembly of fellow addicts. This is every bit as true in the saboteur-driven personality disorders. Here the individual's will is too weakened to resist the internal saboteur and to make the changes necessary to repair the character flaws that generate the saboteur's rampages. But if the individual will is joined to the group will, this becomes a possible, if highly arduous, undertaking. In the process the individual will is strengthened, but more importantly a channel is opened to draw on the power of the collective, universal Spirit-Will.

We must remind ourselves that groups do not automatically form a group will. Rather, the group must be guided into developing its spiritual unity. I have discussed the preconditions for this development in *The Freedom of the Self,* and I elaborate on the general topic of forming a spiritual group in the next chapter and also in chapter 10.

Chapter 6
THE SPIRITUAL GROUP AND OUTPATIENT MILIEU THERAPY

Summary. Despite its obvious advantages in terms of efficient use of personnel and therapeutic power, group therapy is greatly underutilized in US mental health care. The most striking reason is the overemphasis on individual treatment in training programs. Group work is also mistrusted because of its potential to generate destructive mob or antisocial cult misdeeds. Because of its great emotional intensity, spiritual group work, especially when it involves outside socializing, must take special precautions to avoid these outcomes. I trace the origins of my thinking about the necessary safeguards to two experiences in hospital psychiatry, the first during my residency when patients set fire to a psychiatric ward, the second to a milieu therapy unit I ran that initially allowed disturbed patients more freedom than they could handle. What I learned is that a multidimensional program requires an explicit structure in which both staff and patients commit to a shared philosophy of treatment that includes consistent application of criteria for patient admission, staff selection and training, and integrated deployment of multiple techniques to achieve worthwhile treatment goals. In this chapter I show how, with a firm grasp of these principles, a hospital milieu program can be exported and transformed into a spiritualized form of outpatient milieu therapy. When the goals of therapy embody moral-spiritual values, treatment includes but goes beyond symptom alleviation to achieve psychological and spiritual growth, which involves a constructive engagement with community. Its culmination is a life worth living, characterized by development of strong character and the other virtues of leading a moral-spiritual life, not the least of which is making a contribution to the welfare of society—that is, practicing *tikkun olam* (repair of the world in Hebrew).

Group therapy has gotten a bad rap. When invited to join one of my groups, patients typically resist out of fear of having their secret lives exposed to strangers, who might shame them or gossip about them outside the group. Some have already had bad group experiences, from which they have come away feeling that group therapy is an exercise not in self-improvement but in self-indulgence. Others have heard of groups going berserk, even turning into cults.

Since all these unfortunate outcomes can and do in fact occur, the invitation to join a group is not to be given lightly, especially to those who are old hands at other forms of treatment. From the outset, the group leader should take sufficient care to dispel apprehensions by explaining how properly managed groups are rendered safe: by the guarding of confidentiality, the focus on attainable goals, the maintenance of a safe emotional environment, prohibitions against romantic and financial relationships, and the support for nondivisive relationships with patients' families, friends, and social institutions. Cutting off patients from their closest social connections is often the first sign of a cult in the making. Every one of these features of the setup is vitally important.

Once the aforementioned features are understood and agreed to, then the significant advantages of group therapy can be presented. Of all the different forms of psychotherapy, it is the most efficient in utilizing human resources, and more important still, it has the greatest potential for developing the qualities of spiritual healing, for transforming psychological insight and growth into physical and mental inspiration. What follows are some of the considerations that have influenced me in developing a program to realize this potential.

The Structure

Common to most kinds of group therapy is the meeting together of four to eight patients weekly for one to two hours under the guidance of a group leader. The aim of the meetings is for patients to give each other feedback about self-defeating attitudes and behavior. Putting the right kinds of people together and showing them the best way to give feedback are the basic skills of the group therapist. In the first and every subsequent week, patients tell their stories: of failures and triumphs, of being helped or harmed. The other members comment on these narratives, offering sympathy, praise, or critique. If over time the group members come to respect each other and to forge a bond of mutual caring, then the fundamental preconditions are in place for changing the psychological group into a spiritual group: a group that has spiritual healing powers, or put differently, a group that has a strong collective will to health, where goodwill is mutually extended.

My ideas about realizing this possibility have their origins in the psychiatric hospital. I will recount a set of experiences and then draw some conclusions.

The Psychiatric Ward as Microcosm

When I was doing my psychiatric residency in the 1960s, after my Air Force experience mentioned in the first chapter, a catastrophe occurred in what had always been a decorous, tightly organized hospital on Manhattan's Upper East Side. One day, some patients on a locked ward began throwing pieces of furniture at each other. Finally one or two among them piled the furniture in the middle of the dayroom and set fire to it. Firemen with helmets and hoses were soon swarming among suddenly purposeful mental patients.

In retrospect, the conflagration was the culmination of several weeks of increasingly chaotic behavior on the ward: patients had begun to experience more frequent outbursts of anger, sometimes even pushing and shoving each other and screaming at staff members. Nurses had begun complaining that the doctors were undermining their authority and that some of their nursing and social work colleagues were no longer doing their jobs. The emotional temperature on the ward had gotten hotter and hotter, and then on this terrible day, the place had actually burst into flames.

After the blaze was extinguished, the staff postmortems began. How could we as doctors, nurses, aids, and social workers have let things get so far out of hand? Not only was the psychiatric ward wrecked, but patients suffered relapses, with resurgence of previously curbed sick behavior. After several days of intense meetings, we came to some painful conclusions.

For one thing, the admission office had allowed the ward to become populated by a large number of severe "borderline" patients (typically defined as having rapidly shifting identities, moods, memories, and relationships, sometimes with self-mutilation thrown into the mix), who are notorious for being manipulative and unstable and polarizing staff members into warring cliques. Predictably, a faction of the staff had become identified with a group of patients who demanded greater freedom and privileges, whereas other staff members had made common cause with patients who thought the first group was being pampered. According to a prevalent theory about such phenomena, borderline patients typically externalize antagonistic dissociative splits in their own personalities to create warring groups of staff and patients and, outside the treatment situation, friends, family members, and colleagues. The two patient groups ultimately began to toss pieces of furniture at each other, and then the most impulsive and destructive among them bunched the pieces together and set them on fire.

The situation was exacerbated by an ideological struggle between new staff supervisors, adherents of a seemingly permissive form of authority, and an old guard devoted to traditional notions of earned privileges and penalties. In a very important sense, the psychiatric ward had also become a microcosm of this struggle between staff groups. The leader of the new staff, a brilliant researcher who had recently suffered a career setback, arrived on the scene ready for a fight to regain his manhood. He knew he was more competent and clinically astute than his new boss, the head of the department and nominal leader of the old guard. He and his followers took every opportunity to demonstrate that the quality of care the old guard sponsored was seriously deficient and outmoded. In truth, neither leader was very interested in patient care. Neither had sufficient concern for patient welfare to stop their deputies from sacrificing treatment and residency training to their struggle for dominance. Ultimately, the situation was resolved only after the director became ill, the challenger went off to another job, and unified, responsible leadership was brought in.

Lessons and Rules

The lessons to be learned from this debacle are many. It is certainly true that manipulative borderline patients are difficult to treat. In fact they are the bane of the psychiatric facility because of the severity and refractory nature of their destructive symptoms and their capacity to foment conflicts among members of the community. Therefore it is probably unwise to treat more than a few at a time in a small hospital or partial-care unit.

But the most important lesson is that there are essential preconditions for a successful therapeutic program. Certain ideas and procedures, "the rules of the game," and "the treatment philosophy," all of which are expressions of moral values, must be embodied in the daily management of patients.

Otherwise, organizational chaos and symptomatic worsening are likely to follow.

First, the program must have a well-defined, consistent treatment approach. This means that criteria for diagnosing what is wrong with patients are generally agreed on by the clinical supervisors and staff of the program and lead to specific therapeutic interventions with clear goals. For example, using the criteria of the standard nomenclature (now *DSM-V*[55]), all patients diagnosed with major depression are given antidepressant medication and a host of activities designed to externalize aggressive energy and promote activity versus passivity and positive versus negative thinking, until both mood and functional competence are restored or, if possible, are improved beyond pre-illness levels. Other approaches focus on ferreting out early experiences that might have initiated the development of depressive personality features and self-defeating behavior patterns.

Second, the program must have an enunciated philosophy that rationalizes the approach and inspires belief. This is where the all-important moral-spiritual factor either enters explicitly or goes begging. If members of a program come to hold a shared belief system that both dictates an effective, consistent treatment approach and inspires commitment, then the approach will be deployed with the enthusiasm of strong conviction, thereby capturing the all-important inspirational faith factor, often pejoratively termed the placebo effect. The implication is that both the content and the mode of presentation of a treatment philosophy are crucial to its success. For instance, "allaying all symptoms by psychological insight" is not a particularly effective philosophy, no matter how enthusiastically it is presented, as we learned from the disappointing results of the dynamic psychotherapy approach before it was buttressed by biological and cognitive-behavioral techniques. Conversely, psychiatrists who have enthusiasm for either psychoactive medicines or psychotherapy, but not both together, tend to get suboptimal results by objective criteria, at least in the severely mentally ill. (Some cognitive-behavioral therapists dispute this point). Even when the therapist intellectually appreciates the wisdom of a combined approach, just offering it as an objective scientific experiment with no stake in the outcome—that is, not in the inspirational mode discussed in the last chapter—is a strong indicator that the therapist may be best suited for a career in research, not clinical practice.

Third, the program must have an administrative and social process that supports the effectiveness of the approach. The administrative task is to hire staff members who are capable of committing to the belief system and of urging those who cannot to find a more hospitable environment. The same principle applies to the admission and discharge of patients. Totally uncooperative patients are best treated in programs that cater to their range of disturbance; they either should not be admitted in the first place or should be referred elsewhere when they prove unsuitable. The types of patients who meet these exclusionary criteria—paranoid and sociopathic personalities, for example—are discussed later. Most importantly, the treatment philosophy and the program that embodies it must appeal strongly to the hearts and minds of staff and patients. As always, the biggest danger here is that such faith will not be rationally based: that it will derive more from the personal charisma of the supervisors and reverence for their pronouncements than from clear demonstrations of the effectiveness of their approach to treatment.

Social Process

The social process of generating a sense of spiritual mission requires that all patients and staff be members of ongoing discussion groups, involving both education and conflict resolution, devoted to consistently applying the treatment goals and techniques. This must be done in a way that resolves philosophic and procedural clashes and invokes a sense of involvement in a worthwhile cause. As already indicated, the program cannot tolerate irreconcilable conflicts as to the main outlines of the philosophy of treatment or destructive competition among those who run the program. The leadership cannot allow the mission of improving the welfare of patients to be compromised by hidden power struggles and factional splitting. Otherwise, the pathology of the patients is likely to embody an additional social dimension that serves as a microcosm, or hologram, of staff pathology. It is not too large an inferential leap to apply this line of reasoning to the leaders and dependents of dysfunctional families, social movements, and even whole societies.

Before we look more closely at the detailed requirements of such a program, we must tackle the problem of why groups have an inherent tendency to turn destructive. As we just saw, a group of patients influenced by staff discord set fire to a psychiatric ward, undermining its mission of promoting constructive thinking and behaving. How do such things happen?

Mob Psychology

We owe our understanding of the negative potential of group dynamics to the pioneering work of the French anthropologist Gustave LeBon. In his illuminating work *The Crowd*,[56] he elucidated how a mob of ordinary citizens hijacked the French Revolution and turned it into a bloodbath. LeBon maintains that the behavior of the mob represents the lowest common denominator of the personality characteristics of its members. LeBon is saying that minds have the capacity to aggregate, to join together and in so doing to amplify shared mental traits. We might add that those who become the charismatic leaders of such groups tend to embody and express the aggregate's chief passions and aspirations. The personalities of such individuals are, in the sense that I previously defined, holograms or exemplars of the group. In the period around World War II, Hitler was the greatest negative example, embodying the worst aspects of German culture, whereas Churchill was perhaps the finest positive hologram of the stubbornly courageous British people.

Note, however, that LeBon is saying that the aggregation process tends to amplify the most negative qualities of the members of a group. Therefore, one would expect that a crowd of beer-guzzling fans at a sporting event or blind zealots at a political rally could easily turn violent with the right provocation, as indeed we have all witnessed time and again. And this also holds true for the small groups that are involved in social, therapeutic, and spiritual movements, as happened with the cultish addiction program Synanon and the followers of the Indian guru Bhagwan Shree Rajneesh in Oregon some years back. If the leader does not exercise scrupulous control, groups seemingly devoted to good causes can get carried away and indulge in fanatical persecution and wanton sexual exploitation. Mass murder or suicide is the horrific endpoint of such group phenomena, as illustrated by the Waco and Jonestown tragedies and now the suicidal-homicidal terrorist attacks on innocent civilians in all parts of the world by religious extremists. In such cases the aggregation of the most primitive, destructive instincts of the mob, amplified by fundamentalist religious fervor, can culminate in the meaningless destruction of the most cherished values of Western civilization.

Following in the footsteps of LeBon, Freud had a similarly low opinion of groups. In *Group Psychology and the Analysis of the Ego*,[57] Freud in effect says that, as opposed to the more legitimate aspirations of the individual, mass culture always has a destructive thrust. The mass phenomena that make up civilization are included in this sweeping condemnation, as discussed most elaborately in his monograph *Civilizations and Its Discontents.*[58] According to this account, groups are at best repressive, at worst psychotic. One does not have to look much further than this bias to explain Freud's almost exclusive clinical interest in the psychology of the individual, a narrowness of focus from which we workers in the fields of therapy have only recently begun to achieve escape velocity.

When we get away from looking at the world through Freud's narrow keyhole, we discover that groups can also express the *highest* common qualities of their members, not just the lowest. The creation of our imperfect but stable democratic society (for which, ironically, Freud had little affection) by a group of founding fathers, who had to transcend fundamental disagreements, is a happy case in point. Sporting teams that have a winning team spirit that surpasses the talents of individual players; fighting forces that are bold and courageous en masse, even though individual soldiers cringe in their foxholes; the cultural achievements produced by past, sometimes brutal civilizations such as the Roman and British empires—these examples of high common denominators rather than low denominators occur frequently enough that overlooking them attests to the operation of significant biases. Yet we cannot escape the fact that there remains a negative or dark side to spiritual aggregation, usually called evil. I join some theologians in the belief that evil, the "supernatural" antithesis to the good embodied in Spirit, is an ever-present reality that must be taken account of, even used in a limited way, but ultimately guarded against. As we know, power corrupts, and absolute power corrupts absolutely. But we must use it—mindfully.

The Hospital Ward as Therapeutic Milieu

After the ward-burning experience described earlier, I resolved that when the time came for me to administer a hospital program, I would make every effort to maximize the positive common elements and minimize the destructive mob effects of the treatment society. My plan was to implement the principles enunciated previously: a consistent treatment approach, a worked-out treatment philosophy that patients and staff came to believe in, and administrative control over hiring and firing and admission and discharge. My starting point was the concept of milieu therapy as practiced in the 1950s and 1960s, the work of Maxwell Jones, Alfred Stanton and

Morris Schwartz, and a number of group and family therapists who were grappling with how to transcend individual or two-person psychodynamics to understand and harness the larger social forces affecting mental illness and its treatment. My own contribution to this effort was embodied in the program of wards 1b and 2b, the general psychiatric services of University of Wisconsin Hospitals in Madison, which I ran from 1968 to 1972 and described in several publications.[59]

The central idea of milieu therapy is that treatment should be ongoing twenty-four hours a day, seven days a week, not just during the few hours each week devoted to individual therapy sessions. Every encounter with fellow patients and staff members, even chores and recreational time, is to be organized for maximum therapeutic benefit. What I added to this general notion was a technology for implementing it. The rules of implementation were as follows:

1. Have as few rules as possible, only essential ones such as "Patients have to get up for breakfast and attend ward meetings."
2. Combine all effective treatment techniques for each patient: medications plus individual, group, family, and behavioral therapies. When feasible each patient should also be provided with supervised work opportunities.
3. The consistent application of these various approaches has to be ensured by frequent team meetings in which each patient's goals, the means for achieving them, and the level of progress are discussed. To minimize passive attitudes, patients are encouraged to take initiative in designing their own programs and presenting their clinical histories and course in treatment.
4. As mentioned earlier, staff members have to belong to ongoing discussion groups, variously defined as educational or sensitivity-training, to resolve personality conflicts and to ensure a common commitment to the treatment approach—if not with enthusiasm, at least with tolerance for and loyalty to the consensus.

The proper application of these principles leads quite naturally to a treatment program with high morale and a thrust toward clinical improvement. Yet a statement of principles leaves a lot unsaid as to how such a program works. Perhaps some of the missing brushstrokes can be supplied through description of a few untoward clinical experiences and the lessons learned from them.

The Case of the Open Door

Wards 1b and 2b were initially locked wards, and many patients stayed in bed all day, even having their meals served to them. Those who got out of bed tended to congregate in the dayroom watching television or staring off into space. To combat regression, we put patients and nurses in street clothes and got everybody up for breakfast and the daily staff report. Patients were encouraged to take issue with these reports and account for their own behavior. After many hours of staff education, we were able to get everyone to agree that guards on lightbulbs and locked doors only invited patients to find ingenious ways to rebel. So the doors were opened and the lights allowed to shine in their naked splendor. Unfortunately, shortly afterward, one of the most disturbed patients walked out the front door of ward 2b and jumped out the second-floor window onto a flowerbed below, in full view of the hospital CEO, who happened to be passing by. After tending to his sprained ankle, tightening up our supervisory procedures, and eating humble pie in the CEO's office, I (along with the staff) gradually learned to maximize the therapeutic benefit of the open door policy. Other patients helped control access and egress, and free transit had to be earned in stages.

We concluded that greater freedom from social control, and particularly from physical barriers, has to be accompanied by greater attention to their prerequisites, particularly the readiness of patients for fewer restrictions and the readiness of staff for closer monitoring. More generally, all changes in conventional rules must be accompanied by compensatory oversight, preferably in a flexible rather than rigid mode.

Work Therapy and Assertiveness

Another way to combat "hospitalitis," the regressive attitudes induced by chronic hospitalization, is to assign patients to jobs. Not only are they kept active, but they also learn skills that help them lead productive lives outside the hospital. As part of the program, homemakers were taught to grocery shop, to plan menus, and in our experimental kitchen, to cook and serve meals. Some patients were prepared for outside jobs through volunteer positions secured with local businesses and factories. Managers agreed to telephone the patients' teams at the end of workdays and give progress reports, especially about being on time, following directions, cooperating, and meeting deadlines. The willingness of local businesses, such as the Oscar Meyer meatpacking plant, to take part in this program was, to say the least, heartwarming and deserving of expressed gratitude.

One feature of the readiness-for-work program that received special emphasis was assertiveness training. Since many of the patients suffered from depressive illnesses, often characterized by difficulty in deploying aggressive energy, they were helped to role-play situations in which they had to do their jobs and also stand up for themselves. This meant learning not only to take initiative and work hard but also to express their needs and demand respect. Armed with these survival skills, four of the five work-therapy patients were fired in the first week of the program. Typical of the comments sent back to the teams was this one: "He didn't act like a mental patient, more like a lawyer. He was too much trouble."

In our staff review we had to face up to the fact that assertiveness is not an absolute good. Contrary to popular psychology, blowing off steam (or primal screaming) is more likely to do damage than to effect repair. In a culture that has made a fetish of blaming parents for their children's problems, all authority figures are liable to become targets of intemperate complaining. But this is a recipe for failure in the workplace and on the playing field. How things are said and when and to whom are every bit as important as what is said. Assertiveness and honest complaints have to be moderated to take account of social reality. Those in charge have the power to hire and fire and, short of that, to open and close doors. We who were responsible for the ward program had to factor in these considerations. We modified the assertiveness training approach to emphasize courtesy and respect as well as courage in speaking one's mind. Learning to stand one's ground without sacrificing personal integrity or losing composure is one of the most important sets of communication skills, not just in psychiatric treatment, but in every sphere of life. But to confuse assertion with raw anger discharge is to demonstrate a lack of maturity and self-control and to risk causing needless harm to oneself and others. Channeled aggression, the expression of determination and resolve, not name-calling and obscenity-splashing, is the proper goal. We are usually better served by transmuting raw anger into steely determination to do the right thing and to get others to cooperate.

Family Therapy

Under the influence of my colleague Carl Whitaker, a noted family therapist, I initially bought into the family systems theory of symptom formation. As a potent reinforcer of his ideas, Whitaker was often a participant in ward activities, running case conferences and staff sensitivity groups. In his inimitable style, he "fell asleep"—he literally closed his eyes and appeared to be deep in slumber—when he did not like what was going on. What put him into apoplectic coma was the implication that there were biological causes of patients' symptoms or that the root disorder resided in the individual rather than in the whole family system. Yet as much as he hated the idea that we were medicating patients and still holding them individually accountable, he was unfailingly kind and humorous, if not always awake, in his expressions of disapproval. This was a requirement of the expert consultants who helped us apply the various treatment methods that we utilized. They could not, and cannot, be allowed to show ongoing intolerance of different approaches. Otherwise, a multitechnique program in which experts teach their preferred methods to staff and patients collapses under the weight of factional warfare, as we saw in our account of the ward bonfire earlier. Just as our country shows respect for divergent political, religious, and ethnic customs and beliefs, a pluralistic treatment approach must also be integrated, competent, and tolerant of differences.

Family Admissions

In pursuit of the family systems model, we decided to admit family members to the hospital along with the identified patient. Since this was a college community, the family members were almost always the parents and siblings of University of Wisconsin undergraduate and graduate students, most often one or both parents, who were invited to travel from their hometowns to Madison, Wisconsin, and be admitted to the psychiatry ward to join the family member who had become symptomatic. The family took part in all scheduled activities—ward and team meetings—plus group and family therapy sessions. From 1969 to 1972, family members entered the hospital along with the identified patient on roughly 150 occasions.

We were very gratified by the results, which included seemingly rapid symptom relief, an improved sense of family understanding and harmony, and the high morale that comes with the sense of taking part in an innovative, spiritual mission. But in our enthusiasm we failed to notice that we were putting a severe strain on the insurance system that was paying for this expensive hospital care. The effect was comparable, in a bygone time, to expecting insurance carriers to pay for four or five weekly sessions of psychotherapy. Fortunately, by the time Blue Cross discontinued funding the program, we had developed partial-care programs that dispensed with family admissions, so that relatives could participate in the wards' therapeutic activities while staying in nearby motels and apartments. But without the initial experience of twenty-four-hour-a-day contact with patients and their families, it would have been almost impossible to achieve the clarity that we ultimately developed in understanding the role family members play in the genesis or enabling of patients' symptoms and the part they might be asked to play in alleviating them.

Family Impact

With so many different people observing, reporting, and giving feedback on the interaction of many families, ward members were in effect taking a crash course in the social determinants of symptom formation and the opportunities for social remediation. Mindful of the many exceptions and provisos to all such generalizations involving complex human beings and their interactions, we came to the following general conclusions:

1. Some even seemingly cooperative families are so toxic or abusive to their sick members that limited or no contact is the only hope for patients' clinical improvement. Figuring out how to limit contact without generating homicidal and suicidal rage and guilt on all sides—and to still draw on the beneficial resources the family might provide—is no small achievement in these cases. The worst-case scenario, when it is a matter of life and death or recovery versus chronic illness, might involve a permanent cut-off from family members, as illustrated in the last chapter.

2. Parents do not typically *cause* their children to develop major mental illnesses any more than children literally drive their parents crazy. Bad parenting can certainly compromise an individual's future capacity to form good relationships and to live a productive life free of bitterness and self-sabotage. It can also contribute mightily to anxious and depressive lifestyles. But major mood swings, psychotic thinking, and bizarre experiences and

activities are most fruitfully thought of as being fundamentally caused by physical and chemical defects of brain function, commonly of genetic origin, and secondarily by the interaction of these factors with life experiences. Seeing the whole families of identified patients, rather than relying on secondhand reporting, provides convincing testimony to this point. Very often the father, mother, sibling, or child of the symptomatic person manifests a similar clinical syndrome, perhaps different in scope and intensity but unmistakably a variation on the identified patient's presentation. Rigid nurture-versus-nature theorists can always refuse to draw this conclusion and account for comparable (or radically different) personal traits by pointing to the effects of comparable (or dissimilar) rearing conditions. But before there were studies of similarly afflicted children separated at birth and raised apart, the same claims were made on behalf of identical twins with identical diagnoses. In truth, there are enough differences even among identical twins, whether reared together or apart, that neither nature nor nurture alone can do the job. The interactions of nature and nurture must be taken into account, as well as other sources of variance that may as yet be undiscovered.

3. There certainly are different personality types in the same family. When we see many families many times, the two most striking phenomena are the wide range of mental health and sickness in each family and the great differences of opinion among the members as to how the family has functioned to meet its various members' needs. What soon becomes apparent is that well short of mental illness, some children's needs mesh very poorly with their parents' capacities, leading to understandable pain and frustration. Yet other children from the same family paint their childhoods in glowing terms and have high praise for how their parents raised them. Of course, such good matches and mismatches can be discussed exclusively in biogenetic terms, but it is far more fruitful to shift perspectives and look also at the psychological, social, and spiritual factors involved. This allows us to recognize that some parents are temperamentally better suited to caring for some of their children than for others. When parents are controlling and irritable, they are easily provoked by expansive, volatile children. By the same token, calm, caring children can quickly defuse potential blowups and restore emotional balance to the chaotic family. And soothing parents, rather than mercurial ones, do best at pacifying frantic youngsters. Naturally spiritual children are stunted when their mythic-theological explanations are either ridiculed or trivialized by literal-minded family members who have little inkling of a transcendent reality.

At the interface of better and worse matches is where we therapists can do our best work. We try to teach impatient parents to be more calmly supportive and directive, and we show overwhelmed patients how to organize their time and reframe their experiences in ways they were not taught at home or school. Most important of all, we recognize that gender matters. Therapists, parents, and teachers are not temperamentally or sexually or spiritually interchangeable. Sometimes a nurturing mother and at other times a demanding, directive father is what is absolutely required. Therefore, it is desirable to have available a range of teachers and therapists with different temperaments, levels of aggression, depths of spirituality, and degrees of androgyny to meet the individual needs of the enormous variety of patients we see and particularly to show parents and children how to get the best from each other. And we encourage rigidly atheistic parents to tolerate, even enjoy, their children's supernatural musings, especially in a culture so permeated with sci-fi fantasies in film and television.

With these points in mind, we move to the possibility of doing milieu therapy on an outpatient basis.

Group Process in the Outpatient Therapeutic Milieu

The general strategy is to take the principles and practices of inpatient milieu therapy and export them to the outpatient setting. This means that, as much as feasible, the patient's whole waking life is permeated with the therapeutic process. Just as in a hospital milieu, office walls come down, a few relatively firm rules are instituted, and space and time boundaries are flexibly redrawn for specific purposes. Similarly, patients can socialize outside the therapy office for defined goals, such as making observations and giving support and feedback. For this approach to work, the group members must come to share a common belief system about psychological and spiritual growth and the methods for achieving them. Moreover, they cannot be too far apart in age, level of education, severity of illness, and social adaptation. It will not do to mix chaotic teenagers and young adults who have never had a stable career or romantic relationship with successful middle-aged divorcees, or eccentric artists with tightly wound bankers and lawyers. By and large, everyone must be gainfully employed (this includes being a functioning homemaker) or enrolled in an educational program.

These considerations rule out certain types of patients from the outset—such as rigidly paranoid, obsessive-compulsive, addictive, and fanatical (mostly borderline) personality types—because they are all so driven by their needs and fixed ideas that they cannot modify their beliefs and behavior or reliably empathize and show respect and tolerance for those with different character patterns. Antisocial or sociopathic personalities must be ruled out as well because their often charming ways of flouting rules and telling lies virtually guarantee that members of the group will be exploited by them and thereby will lose trust and much more: safety, integrity, and money.

Every group session begins with a short piece of music, such as a Bach prelude, a blues, folk, or rock ballad, or a traditional chant, picked for its special meaning to the leader or members, followed by a joint meditation, which usually takes the form of members visualizing their most eagerly sought outcomes from the program. Outcomes that are predominantly materialistic or egocentric are strongly discouraged in favor of those that benefit the individual and the larger group and society as well. Sometimes these visualizations include best wishes for happy marriages, healthy babies, and recovery from illnesses and social disasters for members of the group. Although visualizations are mostly kept private and discussed in individual sessions, they are at times shared with the group to gain general support.

New patients then tell what difficulties they are experiencing and why they are entering the program, followed by highlights of their past history, family relations, and significant past attempts at treatment. Then veteran members introduce themselves to the new member in similar terms. Analogously to the hospital's daily report, the members give their weekly report: significant progress and setbacks that have occurred since the last meeting, followed by supportive and corrective feedback.

Negative feedback is to be given constructively, in the language of personal reaction rather than moral judgment, and without recourse to deprecation or belligerence. This takes the form of statements such as "You make me feel disrespected when you say I don't know what I'm talking about. How about saying you think I'm not taking account of all the facts?"

Patients who develop irreconcilable differences or destructive rivalries may have to be transferred out of the group if extended efforts at resolution fail. Above all else, the group must have a spiritual atmosphere to do spiritual— that is, creative, healing, and life-affirming—work, and this goal precludes personal struggles that destroy *esprit de corps*, that kill the group's soul. Members must learn to develop a positive attitude, an attitude of hope toward the goals of the program and life in general. Persistent negativity, not less than physical and psychological brutality, is a great enemy of the spiritual life.

The Personal Qualities of the Leader

The leader of a spiritual group must be a spiritual person. Just as the best musicians must be able to realize the numinous (sacred, holy)[60] quality of the best musical scores, the spiritual group leader must be able to recognize and develop the numinous quality of human suffering.

To review the issue once again, we attribute spirituality to individuals who manifest and are moved by Spirit, who exemplify in their own lives the workings of a principle higher than their egocentric interests and outside the spatiotemporal world. The positive aspect of Spirit derives from the linking together of the higher selves residing within each of us: that part of the self that rises above the needs of the empirical, conscious ego. Our higher selves have roots in the universal spiritual stream, or what nineteenth-century writers called the world soul, Bergson called the *élan vital*, and Jung called the collective unconscious. Aggregating the most evolved qualities deriving from these sources constitutes the highest common numerator of a spiritual group. In some hopelessly muddled way, spirit is both *in here* and *out there*—muddled because there is no here *here* or there *there*, for spirit does not reside in ordinary space-time. Yet we mean something important when we say that someone has a soul, is a channel for spiritual energy, or "does the Lord's work." We mean that he or she taps into the common will, the common spiritual stream, and is both a fellow sufferer and a celebrant in serving a higher cause.

In an everyday sense, we know people are spiritual when they can empathize with others in a deep way. Instead of envying a colleague's success or experiencing schadenfreude over his failures, the spiritual person does the work to be able to take pleasure in others' pleasure and to feel pain over their pain, provided that these gains and losses are not purposefully and needlessly achieved at the expense of others. (It is, after all, difficult to empathize with captains of industry who have siphoned off millions of dollars for themselves while driving their companies into bankruptcy and costing thousands of workers their jobs and pensions.) True, the identification is most complete when bridged by an intimate love bond, but the truly spiritual person often feels an intuitive connection even with strangers. Of course, this sense of connection is based on a perception of goodwill and aborts when it is replaced by a recognition of insincere or evil intent.

The leader of a spiritual group must be spiritual in just this sense: able to recognize the higher good in all members and to help them realize it, first by empathizing with their suffering in order to bind it and then by specifically encouraging spiritual repair and growth. This requires a high level of empathic attunement with the feelings, hurts, and strengths of character of each member. Certainly no less should be expected of therapists who aspire to promote spiritual healing. But such therapists will inevitably feel humbled by how far short they always fall in achieving these qualities. We might strive to know all the facts and to be completely effective but must never deceive ourselves into thinking we have reached these goals.

The Education of the Spiritual Healer

Although in some sense spiritual individuals are born and not made, it is also manifestly true that there are large numbers of the latently spiritual who cannot realize this potential in themselves unless they receive the proper exposure to a spiritual mode of being. Encountering mentors who personify these ideals and point the way to realizing them is, of course, the greatest good fortune, expediting the climb to higher realms of experience. Yet there can be no stinting on the hard work of self-development, much of which can be accomplished only in the solitude of disciplined study and exercise, once an accredited mental health training program has been completed. But the understanding yielded by private study must go hand in hand with public engagement. The following are three of the most important principles and practices that inform the work of becoming an effective spiritual therapist:

1. Anti-religious bias must be rooted out because it has no place in the work. Although such a position is understandable in the thought of Freud, who was trying to expunge the irrational and infantile from our thinking about the meaning of life and the possibility of human transcendence, failure to come back around to appreciate the core of spiritual truth common to all the great religions (and the rich heritage they afford, mixed in with their miscarriages) must be regarded as an arrest in psychological and spiritual development resulting in personality constriction. The antidote to this condition involves undertaking specific empathetic and spiritual exercises such as meditation, prayer, chanting, and other consciousness-expanding techniques. These

experiential practices can be profitably introduced and framed by a study of the great philosophers, theologians, comparative religionists, and historians who have probed the essential meaning and universal content of religious and spiritual teachings. At this level, there is no room for intolerance of opposing viewpoints or the kind of literal fundamentalism that claims to have exclusive access to God's mind. This also holds true for secular fundamentalism, which claims to have access to sociopolitical truth without any appreciation of how easily we can be misled by limited information and hidden motivation and the failure to appreciate the realm of supreme values.

2. Just as intolerant atheism has no place in the work, neither do anti-intellectual and anti-cultural biases. To maintain that in times of scarce resources there is no money for art, music, and literature is to betray a philistinism inimical to all spirituality. Once the basic needs of food and shelter and disease control are met, the soul must have its food to survive, and that is what good art and science provide. This means that the truly spiritual person, and especially the spiritual therapist, must cultivate one or more scientific and artistic fields deeply enough to experience their ineffable beauty and truth, in which primitive egoistic gratifications are transcended. Once again, the spiritual therapist, by definition, has great respect for the illumination provided by scientific knowledge. A spirituality that is opposed to scientific progress is misconceived and has to be rethought and deepened.

3. Spiritual therapy in Western society—which values immersion in, rather than retreat from, everyday life—requires that the therapist be tuned into the diversity of popular culture and the major issues of local and world affairs and also be immersed in representative groups that make up the society, particularly those engaged in social repair. Otherwise, the work cannot be sufficiently informed by understanding the particularities of human suffering and deprivation and the potentialities for improvement in contemporary life. This means direct observation of social conditions at all levels of society, both the excesses and the scarcities. It also means wide exposure and appreciation of the most expressive media of our time: cinema and television and the novels, operas, and plays that capture the major spiritual currents of the day and the often dire conditions from which they arise.

Widespread war, crime, and unemployment lend special emphases to the spirituality of the day, as do the comforts of their opposites. Particularly important at this time is some familiarity with the conditions giving rise to the assault on Western humanistic culture by various fundamentalisms. An awareness of present-day concerns about gender definition and identity formation is also mandatory, especially at a time when cultural stereotypes are breaking down. And even if capitalism is the least bad economic system, this is no excuse for failing to recognize the negative impact of unbridled free markets on the individual's search for integrity and universal values, especially when a society places the highest premium on acquisition and winning at all costs. Ideally, spiritual therapists should also have a wide acquaintance with the news of the day by attending to the electronic and print media best known for sound judgment and representation of dissenting opinions. For spirituality to flower, like most meaningful achievements, historical context, with its messy details, must be taken into account.

Anti-Spiritual Pathology

As I have mentioned many times, addictive, paranoid, sociopathic, and severely obsessive-compulsive personalities are the major pathologies that can doom a group's spiritual aspirations. The addict has a prior allegiance, the addictive substance or activity, which precludes an ongoing commitment to a group, its spiritual growth, and the integrity of its individual members. Addicts tend to wash out of all but twelve-step groups, which are specifically geared to transforming their abstinence-indulgence cycles into the more benign addiction to the numerous group meetings. The meeting is the methadone. Otherwise, when the craving is upon them, addicts cannot pay attention to the welfare of loved ones, much less colleagues, and they thereby flunk the major bonding requirement of spiritual group membership. Nor can they be counted on to show up regularly, especially when they are binging. The will of the addict is broken in this special way: it is consumed by craving rather than caring.

Similarly, antisocial personalities, often called sociopaths or psychopaths, are deficient in caring because they cannot see beyond the satisfaction of their own appetites and the avoidance of blame. They have no conscience (a term we use to denote the sense of right and wrong that derives from having the inborn framework for intuiting and developing the values of a common, higher self) to restrain them when their egocentric self-indulgence threatens to cause harm to others. Their presence in a group quickly destroys the mutual trust necessary for therapy programs of any kind, and particularly the spiritual kind. But since blatant sociopathy is rarely encountered in the therapy office, the main concern of the spiritual therapist is its lesser forms: the seemingly ordinary neurotics whose lacunae of conscience are easily missed. What helps to unmask such individuals is their tendency to lie and shade the truth in the service of shirking responsibility. The more materially successful of these mini-psychopaths tend to choose professions that easily lend themselves to the exploitation of others, such as personal injury law and commission sales. This is not to say that there are not ethical practitioners of these fields, only that the temptations these fields afford serve as magnets for the unscrupulous.

The stricture against paranoids is a more complicated matter. We think of paranoia as the tendency to attribute persecutory intent to others where none (or very little on balance) exists. But "paranoia" also applies to unfounded jealousy, which typically involves attributing to the loved one special, often romantic interest in others. Even when these accusations fall far short of delusional intensity, their claimants would tend to destroy the trusting ambience necessary to a spiritual group.

A more insidious problem arises when the symptoms are of only neurotic degree. In these cases bearers of paranoid jealousy are easily mistaken for normally fierce competitors, and their malignant role in undermining a group is underestimated. The tip-off is the persistence of the behavior. No amount of explanation or shared feelings can mitigate the suspicions and accusations that two or more group members express in fighting for the favor of the leader or other desired persons. Sometimes the impasse can be resolved by a better medication regimen, particularly the addition of antipsychotic medications to mood-altering ones. But as mentioned in the last section, such individuals may have to be removed and transferred to settings less reliant on mutual trust.

The paranoid individual, sometimes even when vigorously treated, lacks the potential for true spirituality because the tendency to attribute irreconcilable blame or rivalry to others, the very essence of paranoia, is always divisive. The essence of spirituality, on the other hand, is to overcome divisiveness and join together, to become united with others to make a common cause and form a common self. Because of this hostile divisiveness, the paranoid person cannot develop the empathy to form a spiritual union with others. The paranoid personality is the anti-spiritual personality par excellence.

Forming Spiritual Bonds

Let us be very clear from the outset: spiritual bonds are in large part love bonds. In fact, for many of us, falling in love, supported by the longing for sexual union, is our first and strongest conscious experience of spirituality. Needless to say, such initial attractions do not commonly become fully spiritualized. The experience may be so firmly rooted in sexual passion or the need to dominate or be engulfed that it does not ascend to the higher planes of spiritual love. But just as we presume that all living things have at least a rudimentary form of consciousness, so do we believe that even the most basic kinds of erotic attachment partake of rudimentary spirit, which is at least a partial realization of the desire to unite with and "know" the other person.

We enter the realm of true spiritual bonding when empathic attunement enters the picture. As we shall discuss in a subsequent chapter, empathy comes in many grades. It starts with finding out where other people are "coming from"—that is, what feelings, fears, and fantasies lie beneath their overt behavior and, at a deeper level, what caused these attitudes to develop and what sustains them. Along the way, we come to appreciate their struggles in attempting to rise above their fears and failures. Empathy develops further when the element of caring enters the picture. We go beyond merely knowing where people are coming from and how they got that way to having sympathy for them. We care about their lives, what hand they have been dealt, and how they have played it. Love proper begins when we start to take pleasure in their pleasures and feel pain over their losses, so that their successes fill us with joy and their suffering devastates us. Envy, jealousy, and destructive forms of competition have already been transformed into admiration and emulation: the inspiration to do our best to become as good as those we admire, even to stand on their shoulders to see farther than they do while acknowledging the lift they have given us.

And then that final step of empathic spirituality can be taken. We unite with others to form a common self while still being able to reclaim our individual identity as needed. Spiritual as opposed to neurotic or psychotic union is not a regressive phenomenon. It is not a return to the infant's symbiotic attachment to its mother. It is instead a progressive phenomenon, the achievement of union with the universal soul, the gateway to all-consciousness.

The spiritual group is a therapeutic community, an all-the-time meeting of members who more or less unite spiritually with each other. This means that they come to identify and empathize with and care about each other enough to create a common, higher self that has healing powers for the individuals, the groups they constitute, and the communities around them that share their passion for repair.

Conclusions

A therapeutic group spirit, analogous to the *esprit de corps* of a sports team or military squadron, is generated by putting together patients who have enough self-control to become team players, who can subordinate their egoistic needs to realizing the group's joint project of gaining the most meaningful lives for all its members and the surrounding society. In the process group interaction is extended into the surrounding society, which becomes part of an outpatient therapeutic milieu. This is the highest form of healing possible: people inspired to do their very best because they are connected together in a matrix of mutual caring that also involves the outside world. Just as in a successful hospital therapeutic community, the success of such a venture depends on putting together the right kinds of patients (no addicts, paranoids, or sociopaths); finding a leader who articulates and embodies the spiritual goals of the community (he or she must be an exemplar, a hologram of the group's aspirations); and instituting mechanisms for communicating these goals to the members and monitoring their enactments so that they generate commitment and consistent application. This amounts to placing one's faith in a shared therapeutic belief system about what kind of life is worth living and what is worth doing to get there—in other words, living right. Such commitment is rewarded by the aggregation of a group self that encompasses not the lowest common denominator of a destructive mob, but the highest numerator of a healing circle, the very best in us directed to the enhancement of self, group, and world. In the absence of healthy leadership, such an enterprise, like all emotionally intense undertakings, carries the risk of going out of control and, in the worst case, becoming a destructive cult.

Chapter 7
THE MORAL CODE AND THE SPIRITUAL GROUP

Summary. We can come to know the terms of a universal moral code by virtue of intuition and critical thinking. Our higher self intuits ultimate values, which we must then analyze to determine how best to act on them and how to resolve the conflicts between them. We must concurrently develop the strength of character to will their enactment in our daily lives. In doing so, we can transcend the influences of our bio-evolutionary and experiential backgrounds to make moral judgments and take moral actions that cannot be accounted for and predicted solely in terms of past empirical conditions. The principles of the moral code include prohibitions against murder, abuse, stealing, promise-breaking, and promiscuity; the code also includes exhortations to promote the health and welfare of the poor and dependent, to show gratitude to our benefactors, and to contribute to the repair and improvement of the natural environment. Any spiritual therapy worthy of the name must promote these ultimate values. The spiritualization of treatment can be achieved in individual therapies but is perhaps most fully realized in spiritual groups. Both can promote a caring closeness among participants that can lead to the shared consciousness that forms a higher Self-Will. Care must be taken to ensure that this unification of consciousness transcends but does not annihilate the personalities and freedoms of individuals. Otherwise, intensely connected pairs and groups become susceptible to fanaticism and cult formation. The resulting fervor must be curbed, as previously discussed, by rules and structural qualities that realize the highest common numerator rather than the lowest common denominator of the participants.

There is a universal moral code that all rational human beings can come to know. The principles of this suprapersonal and supracultural code assert that it is wrong to lie, deceive, steal, and cheat; to take unfair advantage, break promises, and betray trust and loyalty; and to inflict mental and physical coercion or harm, commit murder, or worst of all, commit mass murder. Most of these principles are thought to derive from, or at least achieve expression in, the biblical commandments and especially the Golden Rule, which tells us to treat others as we would rationally wish them to treat us. But there are more moral truths in heaven and on earth than can be derived from any single philosophical principle.

The most obvious limitation of the Golden Rule is that it applies most directly to interactive human relationships, leaving the sphere of social rights and obligations less clearly addressed. In this sphere we incur the duties of good citizenship: to support the improvements required to achieve and sustain a just society, one that guarantees the rights of an impartial legal and criminal justice system, socioeconomic mobility, and freedom of expression, assembly, and belief. The just society is charged with protecting all its citizens from unlawful personal and material harm. We as individuals and group members are obliged to work toward ensuring that society embodies these values, while seeing to it that the poor and disadvantaged do not fall through the holes in the social safety net. Repairing these holes pertains especially to providing adequate nutrition, shelter, work opportunities, health care, and education to all. Most commonly we do this by voting for representatives who will fight for these social welfare values and by supporting and participating in the work of organizations devoted to their implementation. But solely as individuals we retain a duty to warn relevant individuals and institutions of society of any impending danger of which we might have specialized knowledge, such as a planned homicide, suicide, or terrorist action, sometimes discovered in an otherwise confidential relationship.

Implied by the foregoing stricture on suicide, the Golden Rule fails to address how we should treat ourselves beyond avoiding irrational and careless self-destruction (smoking cigarettes? bearing unbearable pain?). Ought we not work toward realizing our own highest potential and, indeed, that of all people of goodwill? Shouldn't we preserve and improve the natural environment and the species that share it with us? Rational human beings, with even modest capacities for empathy and rational thought, are likely to answer yes to these questions. They may legitimately disagree, however, as to the most effective means to these ends. People and parties often disagree about resource distribution: for instance, whether resources and work are more efficiently allocated by counting on the "trickle down" effect of favoring wealth accumulation, job creation, and charitable giving by the wealthiest few or whether it should be built up from below by regulations improving the lot of the less fortunate majority who tend to lose out in the competitive struggle of unregulated market capitalism. I believe this a question not of either-or but of both-and, of achieving the right balance between the conflicting values of the two approaches.

Conflicts between Individual Rights and Social Order

As often happens, society's laws impinge on individual rights and freedoms. For example, in the war against terrorism, our government claims the right to monitor private communications and to detain without trial those who are judged to pose a security threat to the larger community. In these cases, currently addressed by the Patriot Act,[61] the individual's rights to privacy and habeas corpus are clearly violated. Yet we might be tempted to weigh in on the side of the government in these cases of conflicting fundamental values because the welfare of the society as a whole sometimes trumps the rights of smaller groups of individuals, at least temporarily in times of great peril. But cases of civil disobedience and conscientious objection continually raise these issues of individual versus group values. And the Golden Rule does not offer much help in deciding these cases, any more than it does in providing a rationale for preemptive aggression or strenuous interrogation techniques of potentially dangerous individuals or groups. Intuitions bolstered by careful assessments of risk-benefit ratios come into play. And compassion for our fellow human beings dissuades us from wanting to kill the murderer, rapist, or potential terrorist, especially since further evidence might prove that we have mistakenly charged or killed an innocent bystander, or a guilty one incapable of acting other than murderously at a particular time but susceptible to rehabilitation in the future.

But there are situations in which we are tempted to reverse our positions after experiencing "teachable moments," in which we discover that we did not foresee the untoward consequences of the actions stemming from faulty moral judgments. An uncritical belief in the innate goodness of all people and their susceptibility to moral rehabilitation is a common source of regrets-in-hindsight that lead to a tougher love of humanity than previously espoused. The only rational course may be to put "mad dogs" away for life.

Take the case of Norman Mailer's support for the infamous Jack Abbott. Abbott, a lifelong violent criminal, was paroled in June 1981, largely because of the advocacy of Mailer and other members of the New York intelligentsia. Abbott had displayed literary talent and lawyerly skills in his critically praised book *In the Belly of the Beast.* In this prison-written tract, he made the case that his past criminal behavior was due to the harsh social conditions of his upbringing and subsequent prison time. Yet only six months after his release from jail, he stabbed a man to death in a New York restaurant over a minor disagreement. Abbott claimed self-defense, but those who witnessed the event saw an individual who could not manage his easily provoked rage. Nor was his next book, once again written in prison, as well received as the first, certainly not by Norman Mailer, who later admitted that his advocacy for Abbott was not among his finer accomplishments.

Cases such as this, coupled with advances in the sciences of genetics and behavior change and a more comprehensive understanding of the causes of immoral and criminal behavior, have rendered obsolete simplistic notions of social conditioning as the preeminent determinant of criminality. To general dismay, the Durham Rule of the mid-twentieth century opened the Pandora's Box of expanding the insanity defense to abrogate or diminish criminal responsibility for any behavior that was judged to be the result of "mental disease or defect."[62] This went far beyond the old standards of individuals' not appreciating the rightness or wrongness of their actions or being in thrall to irresistible impulses. Nowadays we are no longer so ready to make excuses for immoral or illegal behavior—that is, always to reduce bad to mad and thereby render a verdict of not guilty by reason of some degree of mental illness or incompetence or lack of impulse control. Unless external coercion and self-defense can be clearly established, even the manifestly psychotic are more likely to be convicted now than in the middle of the last century.

Other examples of conflicting values are topics of everyday discussion. The rights to choose concerning abortion, contraception, premarital sex, and spousal partners seem, on purely rational terms, to be inalienable rights. But under certain conditions, promoting or exercising these rights as categorical imperatives may not be wise. Taking account of different cultures and belief systems, we might best back off from trying to impose them on traditional religious cultures such as Saudi Arabia and Afghanistan. Yet enlightened Saudis and Afghans have to know that their societies, if they are to continue to prosper, must work toward achieving these fundamental freedoms of choice. In the meanwhile, the controversies evoked by divergent belief systems serve a good purpose. They raise issues of tolerance versus dogmatic belief and flexibility versus feckless lack of character. And they make us engage with the more general issues of how we come to know which principles are absolutely binding and which are only personally preferred or required by law.

Intuition versus Empirical Proof

Kant maintained that we cannot access the principles of the moral law through empirical science because our cognitive processing of sensory data commits us to structuring them only as objects and events causally interacting in space and time.[63] Our brains and their functions, in contrast to our minds and souls, qualify as such spatiotemporal objects causally determined by physical processes. But this spatiotemporal universe never tells us what ought to be or what we ought to do, only what *is* or what is predictable with varying degrees of probability, given our circumstances and past histories. Our commitment to empirical science exhorts us to account for all current phenomena in terms of past conditions and empirical laws, which, if they are the only factors in play, raises serious questions as to whether we ever have free choices and can therefore legitimately be held morally culpable. In giving an unqualified answer to this question, Sam Harris, a well-known neuroscientist and militant atheist, makes the following statement as the premise of his recent book, *Free Will*: "Free will is an illusion. Our wills are simply not of our own making. Thoughts and intentions emerge from background causes of which we are unaware and over which we exert no conscious control."[64]

Where does this leave criminal responsibility? According to Harris, nowhere. Social justice is reduced purely to the practical matter of preventing harm while giving up any notion of morally condemning or punishing the wrongdoer:

> Certain criminals must be incarcerated to prevent them from harming others . . . Dispensing with the illusion of free will allows us to focus on the things that matter—assessing risk, protecting innocent people, deterring crime, etc . . . . Once we recognize that even the most terrifying predators are, in a very real sense, unlucky to be who they are, the logic of hating (as opposed to fearing) them begins to unravel. (op.cit.)

Harris's complete inability, in this case, to think outside the box of spatiotemporal causality is truly astounding. Imagine making such a case to the victims of Jerry Sandusky's predatory attacks at Penn State, or even worse, to the parents of children who have been abducted, raped, and murdered. Unlucky murderers, unlucky victims, unlucky family members, unlucky

Hitler! With Harris's misguided help, we may better "understand" but still not accept what the political theorist Hannah Arendt was trying to say by citing Adolph Eichmann's role in the Holocaust as evidence of what she called "the banality of evil."[65] Evil could be banal only if the perpetrators could not do other than they did because they were just thoughtless cogs in a programmed machine. If this were always the case, then moral condemnation and punishment would never be justifiable, and calling any individual or group evil becomes a mere rhetorical flourish. As Harris would have it, they are just unlucky to be who they are. Sinners that we all are, the same judgment applies to us all.

But such considerations are beside the point once we recognize that the thoughts, beliefs, and commitments that lead to the observance or violations of the moral principles clearly do not entirely reside in the causal empirical world. To be sure, the conditions of child-rearing, education and social indoctrination, and certainly our evolutionary heritage, may interact positively or negatively with the intuitive drivers of our moral beliefs. Yet in their purest form, the universal moral principles are truths residing in a higher, "parallel" universe to which we gain access, partially through the bias-cleansing effects of introspective self-awareness, but most importantly by the faculty of intuition. Tenuously related to Daniel Kahneman's fast thinking and Malcolm Gladwell's blinks,[66] moral intuitions are nonsensory forms of knowing that, to the morally sensitive, appear to be self-evident. The varying degrees of this gift of moral sensitivity, intimately bound up with artistic taste and creativity, can be enhanced or diminished by certain spiritual experiences and practices, already mentioned many times before, among which are conditions favoring or working against the accumulation of human capital.

Enhancers of Human Capital

Human capital, as distinct from economic capital, refers to the knowledge, skills, and personality attributes that lead to success in individual and social terms.[67] These are typically divided into social, intellectual, and health capital. They involve the ability to bond socially, to have the discipline to keep a schedule and complete tasks, to work cooperatively, and to develop the cognitive skills to acquire the information and processing methods to think critically and solve the kinds of problems that lead to productivity. These attributes also include learning appropriate role behavior in the workplace and social situations. These qualities are enhanced by good education, beginning in infancy and early school years and going all the way through high school, college, and postgraduate learning. This educational process at its best emphasizes intellectual curiosity, creative problem solving, and participation in cooperative projects typically involving the sciences, arts, humanities, and sports. Learning to avoid practices that impair health and seeking those that promote a longer, healthier life expectancy are fundamental ingredients of human capital.

There is some evidence that the requisite socialization process begins in infancy. Authorities in the field point to evidence that infants who are regularly and lovingly read to, who are exposed to music and art, who participate in substantive interaction at regular mealtimes or family activities, and who are supervised in tasks and chores—all beginning in the first years of life—are much more likely to develop the discipline, interests, and regularity that ensure the accumulation of large stores of human capital that can be spent throughout a productive life. Moreover, this enriched early family life must continue to involve assignments and obligations until the children and adolescents internalize these skills and values, so that they can be relied on to manifest them on their own initiative. Otherwise, our society breeds an underclass of individuals who cannot secure employment, show up on time, finish assigned tasks, make an effective social presentation, work cooperatively with teammates, care about others, or avoid nonproductive, apathetic, or antisocial behavior patterns such as recreational drug-taking, compulsive TV-watching, and nonstop posting on social media.

Human Capital and Spiritual Values

Put succinctly, high levels of human capital foster the optimal levels of prudence, empathy, inferential reasoning, and intuition that put us in position to gain access to the spiritual realm of universal moral values. By working together and learning to care for and be loyal to each other and to respect social values, we open the door to realizing that we share a common spiritual being and therefore a common fate. This one-mindedness can be developed further by age-old spiritual practices, including various forms of meditation, prayer, yoga, and martial arts, all done with the goal of transcending individual consciousness to reach the realm of spiritual awareness, wherein resides the

Spirit-Will of a common Self that stands for and manifests what is universally true and good.

Illusions and Moral Conflicts

Unfortunately, as we all must recognize, our intuitions are fallible. We are led astray by the usual suspects: deficient human capital from bad genetic makeup and inadequate upbringing, neurotic needs often involving primitive narcissism, biases inculcated by parochial social conditioning, and irrational, sometimes psychotic, thinking taking the forms of illogic, paranoia, grandiosity, and absolutist intolerance. The contamination of intuitions, which can lead to illusions if not downright delusions, places a heavy burden on all people of goodwill who have no other recourse than cautiously trusting the intuitive faculty in everyday encounters with the seen, the unseen, and the unforeseen. So we must carefully check the validity of our intuitive beliefs by subjecting them to rigorous self-scrutiny and to the scrutiny of our most trusted friends and colleagues and, of course, by repeatedly checking for sources of misjudgment and the unintended consequences of our actions.

As if these obstacles to truth were not sufficiently daunting, we also frequently find ourselves—we say it yet again—in situations where our moral principles are in conflict, so that we must choose to follow one in violation of others. We must kill another living creature in order to ensure our own survival and that of our loved ones and our group. Our loyalty to one individual or group is purchased at the painful cost of disloyalty to others to whom we are also indebted. An important consequence of such conflicts is that they often lead to the mistaken impression that there are no abiding values, only situationally relevant ones. The more tragic truth is that in resolving such conflicts, we are forced to bite into the bitter fruit of knowledge that we cannot escape doing wrong, no matter how conscientiously we try to lead a moral life. We are reduced to trying to do the least harm possible given the options at our disposal. Making accurate calculations about more or less beneficial or adverse consequences in these cases requires the most careful examination of empirical and spiritual influences and their interactions. These determinations constitute the essence of critical thinking.

Critical Thinking

Confronted with cloudy or conflicting loyalties and beliefs, we must clarify and focus our thinking to determine whether our moral enthusiasms and indignations are founded on base motives such as jealousy and greed rather than ideals of fairness and caring generosity. And we must come up with best estimates of the various consequences of alternative courses of action. In these calculations we can sometimes think in simple utilitarian terms—to achieve the greatest good for the greatest number—but such widespread goods cannot come at the expense of causing suffering to even small numbers of innocent children, poor and disabled victims, and disenfranchised minority groups. Above all, we must try by all means to avoid using the fate of certain individuals to further the interests of ourselves or favored others, for in so doing we violate the fundamental Kantian notion that we must treat all people as ends in themselves, not as means to furthering our exclusive interests. It is not just attorneys and physicians who are obligated to have a fiduciary relationship with their clients. We all must strive to have a fiduciary relationship with each other, so that we balance our own gains and losses with their consequences for others.

By such critical thinking we refine our intuitions to formulate valid principles of the moral code. In so doing we maintain that these values are "objectively" and universally good even though their validity is not typically provable by scientific evidence and even though they do not always come in a straight line from our first intuitions.

Morality and the Anomalous Position of Psychotherapy

Ironically, the field of psychotherapy, especially in its popular psychodynamic and behavioral forms, seems to dissent from the position that moral truths exist and are knowable, much less that they should be used to shape our therapeutic interventions. We practitioners often come off as standing for moral neutrality or, at best, moral relativism. In fact, by giving preeminent roles to inborn constitution, motives, and conditioning in explaining human behavior, psychotherapists influenced by the theory of psychic determinism typically call into question the legitimacy of making overt moral judgments about patients and directly or indirectly inducing them to reform. Rather, we typically place preponderant emphasis on understanding the causes of symptomatic behaviors rather than judging their moral value. We become preoccupied with *why*, in terms of past conditions, patients do what they do rather than precisely *what* they do to themselves or others and what they ought to do or not do. In the process we accord little or no significance to the moral worth of our patients' actions, much less our own. Actions become not so much good or bad but more or less explainable. There is no doubt that pretending to such a value-free position has its strategic uses: the implicit acceptance of bad behavior encourages patients to confide in us, to speak openly of their failures and transgressions, thereby lessening guilt and opening up the possibilities of new insights, better behavior, and greater trust in our goodwill. Yet we cannot expect them to find a better life if we do not represent and encourage better, more productive values than those they have brought to treatment. In the process, we have a chance to help them transform old inadequate guiding principles into a spiritual value system. We might open a door that, with hard work and no small amount of luck, can lead to a more creative, meaningful, and fulfilling life.

So with no apologies for making assumptions that run counter to the stripped-down values of mainstream schools of therapy, I propose the following list as the main terms of a modern humanistic and spiritual moral code, one that is meant to serve as a guide to therapists and patients alike for learning to lead a fulfilling life of moral integrity:

Do not kill except to neutralize existential threats.

Do not steal, lie, or cheat except in rare cases of avoiding social catastrophe.

Keep your promises except when bad consequences trump the loss of trust.

Do not physically, sexually, or psychologically abuse others.

Do not engage in incestuous or power-imbalanced intimacies.

Avoid emotional and sexual promiscuity.

Preserve and improve the environment and its life forms.

Care for poor, disabled, elderly, and dependent human beings.

Be loyal to parents, loved ones, mentors, and colleagues short of their betrayal of trust.

Develop one's potential to the fullest and promote the development of others.

Contribute services and capital to causes that promote the rights of individuals and minorities and the common good.

Warn others of clear and impending catastrophic dangers.

Clearly, more provisos might be appended to these principles, and some may have higher priority than others in situations of conflict. In addition, each may need critical examples and more precise definitions to operationalize their usage. These may be found in the writings of our greatest moral philosophers and, not to be overlooked, the novels of the great masters of the form. On a less exalted level, columns such as "The Ethicist" in the Sunday magazine of the *New York Times* offer many everyday moral dilemmas and their proposed resolution. Chosen at random, I offer the following exchange from "The Ethicist," between a reader and the columnist, as a typical example.[68]

> *Five years ago my dear friend **A** was [devastated] when her husband asked for a divorce. Now just . . . after her divorce was finalized, she has met an old boyfriend who is married to [my acquaintance] **B**.*
>
> ***A** . . . will be married to this old boyfriend [who] plans to announce to his wife [**B**] that he wants a divorce. **B** . . . is completely unaware of the impending disaster . . .*
>
> *[Of] several roads to travel here: one is to confront **A** and*

remind her of her [past] pain . . . Another option is warning
***B** . . . A third is to keep my mouth shut . . . Am I ethically*
*obligated to admonish **A** or warn **B**?*

The first part of your query is simple: You should confront **A** and force her to consider what's going to happen when she does this. I would be surprised if your admonishment had any impact, but it's still a necessary conversation . . .

The second part . . . is more intricate: are we ethically obligated to warn other people whenever we recognize an imminent danger they cannot see themselves? . . . What you need to reconcile is your relationship with **A**. If she's truly a close friend (and will remain such . . .) you should not intercede with **B** . . . [A] doesn't pose a physical threat to anyone, or to herself. She's telling you this because she trusts you . . . and wants your input . . . . Tell **A** that you disagree with what she's doing and that her behavior will alter the way you view her character. Allow her to explain why she entered a relationship with a married man . . . . Remind her that **B** is going to feel the same way she did five years ago. But don't blow up your friendship because someone pursued a romance you find abhorrent. Humans make mistakes.

This example, whose conclusions are questionable, vividly illustrates the complexity of moral decision making when fundamental values are in conflict and, more specifically, when the terms of the discussion are not carefully defined. Among those values in conflict are the loyalty owed a friend versus an acquaintance and how this affects the conflict between the duty to warn and the duty to be loyal to and forgiving of loved ones. Also, the term "danger" covers many possibilities: hurt feelings, physical harm, and death of the soul or the body. The ethical advice-giver in this case placed the highest value on preserving a deep friendship over behavior that cannot entirely be morally justified but that falls short of inflicting physical harm, which is obviously regarded more seriously than the psychological harm of devastated feelings. This may well be an underestimation of the impending damage. What if **B** becomes suicidal following the betrayal? Shouldn't that possibility of physical harm have been considered?

Note, however, that both the ethicist here and most others who come to grips with the morality of everyday life inevitably assume the existence of enduring values, even as they try to resolve the conflicts between them and to clear up the murkiness of the terms of the discussion. Although most thinking people try to avoid speaking of these values in absolutist terms, I have tried to be explicit about them and will continue to do so, even though critical thinking may alter how I choose to formulate and act on them in specific situations.

Advocacy and What It Entails

By advocating a moral-spiritual therapy, I mean to take every opportunity to encourage the expansion of consciousness in students and patients that leads to moral behavior. It does not mean that I am forever scolding and cajoling to get myself and others to do the right thing. I try not to weigh in on cases of nickel-and-dime morality such as minor, occasional misdemeanors that are unlikely to do permanent, serious damage to the character of perpetrators or the welfare of their victims. And however distasteful I might find playing endless games of solitaire or fantasy ballgames, I do not think it worthwhile to dissuade patients from these relatively harmless activities.

But I do advocate setting limits on instances of severe destructive behavior and encouraging better alternatives. As I discussed in a prior publication,[69] setting limits attempts to dissuade individuals and groups from taking what are judged to be immoral or destructive courses of action, by raising questions as to their prudence, by painting vivid pictures of their potentially untoward consequences, and by appealing to patients' will to health, security, and common decency. If these measures are unsuccessful, then I (and other like-minded therapists) may choose to express stronger forms of disapproval. These may go all the way from threatening loss of respect to dissolving the therapeutic relationship and, of course, exercising the duty to warn loved ones, potential victims, and if necessary, law enforcement agencies when lethal danger to self or others is imminent.

Implications of Moral-Spiritual Truth

The principles embodied in these rules are the main constituents of the moral code and are basic to leading a spiritual life. Breaking any one of them frays one's connection to Spirit, to our common consciousness, and murdering the innocent severs it completely, resulting in the loss of Soul, often permanently. The light goes out in the eyes, and the heart grows cold. Even soldiers serving a humanitarian cause find it difficult to shake off the soul-altering effects of their kills. At the deepest spiritual level, the moral principles are justified by our intuition that we and our world have a common Soul. We share a common consciousness, even though we may not always be aware of this reality. Individual minds are constituents, microcosms, or holograms of an all-embracing Mind-Spirit-Will in which each of us can and should strive to participate. Vitality and caring are among the signs of success.

The unity of consciousness sets the task for spiritual growth and healing: we must do the work of attaining the higher awareness that enables us to be identified and unified with the one overall consciousness. Once we gain the awareness that our individual souls are parts of a larger whole, known variously as Soul, Spirit, Self, Will, Life Force, or God, all the rules of the code naturally follow. They all involve loving and being good to oneself, and therefore to one Self. Violating any one of them is tantamount to attacking one's own being. Harming another is harming the Self. Even if we are compelled to destroy genocidal maniacs such as Hitler or Pol Pot, we are doing nothing less than cutting out a cancer of the common Soul. In the process, we experience not narcissistic self-injury but Self-injury. We prune the tree of life so that it may recover from a cancerous or diseased growth and become stronger. But it would be foolish to think that the pruning does not take a toll. Ask the German and Austrian people what ridding themselves of Hitler and his regime cost the lands of Bach, Goethe, Kant, Mozart, and Beethoven; and think of the spiritual patrimony lost by forcing the exile of geniuses such as Mann, Einstein, and Freud. Almost seventy years later, the despoiled soil of German culture has only now begun to bear shoots of its past fertility.[70]

Once again, one of the greatest obstacles to following the moral principles is that they often stand in conflict. There are circumstances in which violating one rule may be required to avoid violating another to which we give a higher priority. For example, we choose to shade the truth to avoid delivering a devastating blow to someone's self-esteem ("Given your past history, you couldn't help fleeing the scene of the accident"). For this and other pragmatic reasons, Mark Twain (1835-1910) said we dare not tell the whole truth except in our private diaries, not to see the light of day until long after we and our contemporaries are dead. As he wished, his diary has only recently been published, one hundred years after his death.[71]

In making this point, I do not mean to blur the distinction between right and wrong. Rather, by acknowledging ambiguities and exceptions to doing the good, we gain greater awareness of moral complexity. One of the most poignant testaments to both moral awareness and moral exception occurs at the end of Saul Bellow's novel *Mr. Sammler's Planet.* The main character, a highly cultured refugee from Nazi Germany, arrives at the morgue and delivers a prayerful eulogy over the body of his nephew Elya, a physician who, despite his criminal enterprises, was generous and loyal in his personal life.

> Remember, God, the soul of Elya Gruner, who, as willingly as possible and as well as he was able, and even to an intolerable point, and even in suffocation, and even as death was coming, was eager, even childishly perhaps (may I be forgiven for this), even with a certain servility, to do what was required of him. At his best this man was much kinder than at my very best I have ever been or could ever be. He was aware that he must meet, and he did meet—through all the confusion and degraded clowning of this life through which we are speeding—he did meet the terms of his contract. The terms which, in his inmost heart, each man knows. As I know mine. As all know. For that is the truth of it—that we all know . . . [72]

We *do* know. We know the moral law within. Through our true self's connection to Spirit, we gain the intuitive knowledge that informs the moral code. But there is more to it. The evolution of the human species has ensured that we have a biological infrastructure on which to hang this intuitive awareness; it consists of the survival mechanisms embedded in our genetic material by the evolutionary process.[73] Yet becoming aware of and acting on the moral laws is subject to confusion and doubt. Growth in spiritual awareness helps us find a way through the "cloud of unknowing." The greater our spiritual wisdom, typically earned by suffering losses and failures in our life, the better our chances of finding the path to a life of meaning and worth. I say "wisdom" instead of "information" or "knowledge" because wisdom attaches to the highest forms of truth. It is knowledge that has been evaluated for its potential to contribute to personal integrity and the common good. Achieving spiritual awareness is a necessary precondition of gaining wisdom. Information, in contrast, is about facts and bits: the transmissible data accessible to ordinary empirical consciousness. Ordinary knowledge derives from the ability to place observable facts within a coherent conceptual scheme that has been screened for bias. As to wisdom, this is what Bellow says we know—or can and should know. It is the spiritualized knowledge that tells us what is *worth* knowing and doing and what kind of life is *worth* living.

The Issue of Making Amends

There is no getting around the fact that trying to make amends is often impossible. Despite its central role in twelve-step programs such as Alcoholics Anonymous, attempts to apologize and make up for past misdeeds can misfire, opening up old wounds that are best left to scar and heal as best they can. Birth parents who have put up infants for adoption should not always, from a position of greater spiritual maturity, try to locate them in order to make amends. When these well-intentioned fantasies for reconciliation result in dashed hopes, additional psychic damage, rather than healing, can be the result. The same is true of the reverse situation, when adoptees search out their birth parents, only to find them unrepentant and unable to express the love and sense of loss that had been hoped for. My patient Paula, suffering in midlife from poor health attributable in part to early abandonment, found not only a cold, rejecting birth mother, but one who had abandoned yet another child. Although she gained some compensation by making contact with and befriending this newly discovered half sibling, she still suffered serious relapses in her mental and physical illnesses directly following the devastation of contacting her biological mother.

Do No Harm

Yet we can learn from these often misguided attempts. By way of illustration, I want to describe an experience in which my misconception of the possibilities for making amends led me to break the physician's solemn oath to do no harm. I have discussed this case in an earlier work, *The Freedom of the Self* (1993). I will review it again here and spell out some of the knowledge and hoped-for wisdom that I may have gained as the years have passed.

John, a twenty-seven-year-old health care worker, consulted me for depression. Eight years earlier, he had been drinking in a bar with his girlfriend. Afterward, in a rainstorm, they had driven home, exceeded the speed limit and run over two people in a crosswalk. His girlfriend begged him to stop, but John stepped on the gas pedal. As a result of shared guilt and recriminations, their relationship fell apart soon afterward. Now eight years later, he still felt tormented by his actions. In the days following the hit-and-run, he discovered from the radio that he had collided with a newly married couple and that the wife had died in the hospital, but the husband had managed to survive. According to the newspapers, the police held a suspect in custody. John never read the papers or listened to the news again. He tried to assuage his guilt by taking a job in health care.

In the course of our attempts to understand his predicament, he got in touch with a previously split-off memory. When John was around age ten, while his parents were out of town, his older brother Mark, with whom he had been wrestling in a swimming pool, suddenly turned blue and died. Family happiness was never regained. Even though his parents tried to absolve John by revealing that Mark had suffered from a congenital heart defect, he felt responsible for his brother's death and the purported ruin of the family.

On antidepressant medication and weekly therapy, John improved somewhat but not enough to feel good about himself. At the time, much of the discussion in the ethics and psychiatry literature took exception to the stance of moral neutrality recommended by most schools of mental health treatment. In the interests of pursuing a more comprehensive therapy, some teachers urged their clinician-trainees to hold patients morally accountable for egregious misdeeds. Making amends, it was suggested, might be the pathway to regaining moral integrity with its attendant therapeutic benefits. This kind of thinking led me to push John to examine the prospects for making amends for what he had done.

What would happen if he turned himself in? What if he contacted the surviving husband and put himself at his mercy? What had happened to the suspect in custody? The good news was that the suspect had been let go for insufficient evidence. But all the other avenues for amends proved to be dead ends. The law was in no position either to punish or to absolve him at this late date. The husband had remarried and apparently moved on with his life. Stymied but pushed by me, John felt increasingly frustrated and demoralized. Before long, he dropped out of treatment altogether, certainly in no better shape, probably worse, than when he began. So much for my physician's oath, *primum non nocere*—above all else, do no harm.

Treatment When Amends Cannot Be Made

Among the many issues that this case brings up is that redemption cannot always be fully and feasibly achieved. There are misdeeds or crimes that are so immensely destructive that making amends is not only impossible but also virtually irrelevant. The wanton murder of innocent schoolchildren leaves a stain on the monster's moral fabric that can never be scrubbed clean. Because the murderer may have been afflicted by some disorder that affected judgment and impulse control, he might be absolved of criminal responsibility, but he can make no apology or repayment that would suffice in the purely moral-spiritual realm. An orthodox religion that dispenses full absolution might be of more help here than spiritual therapy. In John's case, the time for making amends had already passed. But this was no reason not to offer him spiritual therapy involving assuagement of guilt and help in discovering reasons to go on with his life. He needed to be "forgiven" in the form of understanding and acceptance by me in order for him to grant a measure of forgiveness to himself. Then he might possibly lead a less depressed, more meaningful life, despite harboring a black mark inside. Perhaps he could lighten the mark by soldiering in the trenches of good works.

The assumption here is that true absolution in the religious sense is not in the repertoire of the secular or the nonreligious spiritual therapist. Giving absolution, if it can be done, is the domain of priests and shamans, not therapists or counselors. But if we are spiritual beings who realize that we are all sinners, then we should not make life harder for our fellow transgressors by piling on when they are already down. What John needed from me, a professional helper, and above all from a supportive group was a measure of comfort and acceptance, not more impossible tasks to perform that emphasized how sinful he had been. He needed to know that, in my opinion and the opinion of a group of fellow sufferers, there were forces beyond his power to resist that had caused him to hit-and-run. We could offer up these factors to diminish his sense of guilt and his otherwise soul-crushing moral devastation. His behavior was perhaps conditioned by the early traumatic death of his brother, for which he felt so overwhelmingly guilty that he had initially had to split off the memory in order not to come apart. To give him the benefit of the doubt, a group and I might have argued that taking full responsibility for his drinking and negligent driving by calling the police and an ambulance would have once more threatened to tear him to pieces. To protect himself, he had physically split as he had previously mentally split.

It was his defensive or coping style. This characteristic behavior indicated a character deficit that he needed to arm himself against in the future—as another patient, Ned, did after owning some responsibility for the death of his son (discussed in chapter 8)—but he did not need to continue to torture himself for his behavior in the past. If I had helped him accept his limitations, then he might have found a way to transcend some of the burden of living with his character flaws.

The Possibility of Lesser Amends

Fortunately, there is a more forgiving possibility. Not infrequently we commit offenses of a less ruinous nature that we can and should make amends for. The violations of the moral code short of premeditated or impulsive murder are all, in favorable circumstances, viable candidates for remediation. There are also the everyday nickel-and-dime mishaps. When we bang into a parked, unoccupied automobile, we should leave our telephone number and assume responsibility for repairs. Since all is *not* fair in love and war or in the skirmishes of free-market capitalism, we can and should make amends for overcharging or underpaying a friend, client, or business establishment. Nor should we enter into marriages or other contracts and covenants without revealing skeletons in the medical or legal closet. Having an undisclosed chronic illness or genetic defect stands a significant chance of fostering an unhappy marriage and an even unhappier, impaired child. All proposals of marriage or employment should come with disclosures of past brushes with the law and past illnesses of consequence. Otherwise, the consent to enter into the contract by the other party cannot be rationally informed. Out of shame and fear, many people withhold vital information, but the failure to come clean can have serious aftereffects.

As a case in point, a prominent professional man, known for his volunteer work on an international scale, neglected to tell his fiancée that he had virtually no ordinary income or savings. He lived off the expense reimbursements, generously enhanced, afforded by the organizations sponsoring his volunteer work. After marriage, the truth came out when they met with an accountant for tax advice. The bride discovered that she had possibly taken on a financial and emotional burden she had not counted on. Had she known what she was getting into, she might have made other choices and been spared the resentment that wormed its way into the core of the marriage. Yet with some imagination and courage, many such misdeeds can be made good on, in the process generating stronger trust and commitment between those involved than had existed before. In this case, the full-time volunteer made sufficient amends—involving greater transparency about his affairs and lightening up on his volunteer work to make a good-faith effort to resurrect his private professional practice—to salvage what turned out to be a reasonably good marriage.

Making Good on Losses

Beyond misdeeds, there are losses that one can never entirely repair. Ask any parent who has lost a child or a beloved partner, or children who have lost parents or siblings before their time. The gaping hole in one's being, encompassing both self and Self, is ever present. But just as we can, if we are blessed, provide good enough care to our children so that they can face the world with a basic sense of security, so we can as therapists and colleagues provide good enough support to help those with irreparable losses and past transgressions to go on living. It is not too much to hope that we can provide the support and guidance that will lead them to repair the self by contributing to the repair of the world, thereby coming closer to balancing the moral ledger of the greater Self. It helps if the method of repair bears a vital relationship to the earlier loss, such as working in an AIDS care facility if one has lost a son, sibling, or partner to the disease or working with organizations that try to find missing children if one's own child was fatally abducted.

Making repairs for losses is obviously not the same as making amends for moral or criminal misdeeds. But at their gravest, they have this issue in common: they both involve an irreplaceable loss, in the one case loss of the integrity of the self, in the other loss of a treasured relationship belonging to the common Self—in other words, the loss of a true love relationship, one that transcends egocentric needs. They both qualify as perhaps the worst calamities that can befall human beings, threatening the continued existence of our humanness, of having a soul. They put to the test our ability to transcend losses to continue living a meaningful, fruitful life. The outer limits of this possibility occur when we have impulsively sacrificed the life of another person, especially a loved one, in order to save our own. Those who put others in the position of having to make this choice, as the Nazis did in the concentration camps, know that there is little life worthy of the name left to the survivor without superhuman efforts to wall off the experiences from consciousness. No excuses, such as being betrayed by our instinct for survival, will let us off the hook. Perhaps this is the place for religious absolution or for achieving that mystical or Nietzschean state that is alleged to lie beyond good and evil.

The Moral Code for Therapy

How do we ensure that we follow the moral code in doing psychiatric treatment and psychotherapy? We do this by offering not merely medical and psychological treatment, but moral-spiritual care. We begin by manifesting a genuinely caring attitude and making a mighty effort to empathize fully with the suffering of those who seek our help. But spiritual care goes beyond this. Based as it is on the awareness that therapists and patients share a common consciousness, therapy must be offered exactly as empathetically caring therapists would want to be treated if they were in the patient role. Therapy must be offered not in a harsh, negative way, but in a maximizing, positive one. To avoid misunderstanding, I do not mean to exclude from this approach the tough love that might be required to reverse a destructive personality trend such as philandering and narcotics addiction.

Caring, whether tough or tender, is still caring. Concurrently, the same care should be required of patients. They should be helped to treat the therapist and others with the same regard and consideration that they would rationally want for themselves, increasingly learning to intuit and understand their common human needs and aspirations and their special ones as well. This is an essential feature of all psychological and spiritual growth, the aims of psychotherapy beyond symptom relief. If the rest ought to follow naturally, the therapist may still have to take the lead in making certain that therapist and patient do not abuse or exploit each other, financially, physically, or emotionally. Beyond this call of duty, those of us who treat actively suicidal or borderline psychotic outpatients, along with others with special needs, know that they may have to be given direct access to us in times of crisis, no matter how disruptive of our schedules or private lives this may prove to be. Since many of these patients have been emotionally abused or abandoned by cruel or detached parents, these crises provide an opportunity to provide the caring identifications—the personalized support, empathy, and limits—that engender the love of self and the surrounding world that make us feel blessed to be alive. In this way, the path is cleared for the life force, the will to life, to inspire us to become creative and healing rather than negative and destructive.

Therapists who cannot or do not choose to be fully available to patients in crisis might do well to restrict their practices to less demanding patients. As a longtime supervisor of medical and nonmedical mental health trainees, it has been my experience that sometimes they are carelessly assigned patients who are teetering over an abyss, whom they are not prepared to rescue. All too often, suicide attempts and psychotic decompensations are the consequences of these mismatches. Because of either temperament or lack of experience, these budding therapists—I count myself as having been one of them—do not recognize when desperate people are truly desperate and thus need immediate lifesaving or soul-saving attention. We know of patients who have gone into a suicidal or homicidal rage after they have made one final effort to reach out for help, only to be sternly rebuffed by therapists or "friends" who reprimand them for disturbing their sleep or for manifesting "weakness of will."

Implicit in this discussion is that spiritual therapists must tune into the spiritual potential as well as the spiritual needs of their patients and help bring them to repair and fruition. Uncommon sensitivity to the needs of others, spontaneous acts of charity, lifestyles that manifest moral rather than materialistic values—these must all be recognized and reinforced in our patients as well as ourselves, especially when these qualities go largely unappreciated in the everyday world. Most important of all, since spiritual therapists are spiritual by virtue of striving for integrity of character and highly attuned empathy with the plight of others, then we must earn the privilege of serving as role models for patients by manifesting the very qualities ourselves that we wish to help strengthen in them.

The Spiritual Dimension of the Outpatient Milieu

The application of the moral and spiritual perspective is intrinsic to developing and maintaining an outpatient therapeutic community, as I have defined it. At its best, such a community makes the moral rules present and real for its members. And it does this by providing the conditions for their achieving spiritual awareness. It enables the members to appreciate and treat each other not as means to their own ends, but as ends in themselves. In others words they have the opportunity in the spiritual group to learn to truly care for others rather than use them mainly for their own purposes. In this way the moral code becomes manifest in their relationships with each other and indeed with the world as a whole. Spiritual awareness tells us that "I" and "Thou," at the deepest level, are one and the same; moreover, the empirical world outside us, the "that" of sensory perception, is the same "stuff" as the "I." As some of our greatest thinkers have realized, the world is less like a great machine and more like the great thought or dream of an all-encompassing mind, and this dream is permeated with the ultimate spiritual values of caring, truth, and goodness, which has the potential for overriding the misery and decay that we also see around us.[74]

This squeezing together of the teachings of Martin Buber, the Upanishads, and quantum theory gives us the fundamental truths of the Spirit: that the reality behind the observable world is willful consciousness or Spirit and that this willful consciousness is all of a piece. Typically, we have immediate experience of these truths only fleetingly and dimly. When they are more firmly grasped and go on to permeate a whole group, then the members experience "mutually assured ego-destruction" temporarily. The self-interested self or ego gives way to the Self-interested Self, whose wisdom tells us that we must be one for all and all for one. Achieving this unitary consciousness gives us intuitively the universal moral principles, the wisdom to know what to value most and therefore how to act. Acquiring this wisdom in the depths of our being gives us our main chance of finding the great peace and joy that exists right here in the all-encompassing now, the goal of all great spiritual teachings.

Group Consciousness

The spiritual group provides a unique opportunity for its members to progress toward developing a unitary, spiritual consciousness. We have already spoken of many of the preconditions: the membership cannot include members who are rabidly destructive of group cohesion, such as sociopathic and paranoid personalities; disruptive conflicts between members must be quickly resolved, even at the expense of discharging the participating parties; and the leaders of such groups must exemplify spiritual striving in the way they lead their lives, particularly in treating everyone fairly and encouraging the nascent spiritual qualities of the members and, in favorable circumstances, everyone they encounter in their daily lives. But meeting such preconditions, though necessary, is not sufficient to spiritualize a group. The members must also develop a high intensity of feeling for each other and for the group enterprise as a whole.

Spiritualizing the marital bond is catalyzed by achievement of a joyous and mutually penetrating sexual union. But in therapy groups, sexual liaisons as well as projects involving monetary exchanges between the members are rigidly proscribed because they expose the members to heightened risks of divisiveness arising from jealousy, subgrouping, and perceived harm. If these sources of conflict are not dealt with forthrightly but rather are sealed over by formulaic rituals and loosey-goosey protestations of "love," the group is likely to take on the characteristics of a cult, with disastrous consequences not only for the group itself but also for the surrounding society. Witness the Branch Davidian massacre in Waco, Texas, in 1993, tied to sexual exploitation by its leader David Koresh and a botched FBI intervention; and the financial exploitations of the Shree Baghwan Rajneesh cult in Oregon, evidenced by the leader's numerous Rolls Royce sedans, paid for by members' contributions and the possession of which Baghwan termed a "cosmic joke." Some joke! What then do we substitute for sexual union or extra-therapy causes and projects as a means of intensifying group relations to the point of spiritual bonding?

Breaking a Conventional Therapy Rule

I have found that allowing members to socialize with each other outside the group, even though unconventional, is an effective way to do this. As a result group members become intensely interconnected and have a better chance of developing a group spirit. This is as true of basketball teams and string quartets as of therapy groups. All these groups can function as wholes greater than their parts when the members come to care about each other enough to hang out with each other as an adjunct to their joint commitment to a common mission. Sheer technical proficiency will not do it. A group of all-stars will not win a sports championship if they lack chemistry and rely only on individual proficiency.

For example, the chemistry born of trust and caring broke down between quarterback Donovan McNabb, tight end Terrell Owens, and the 2005 Philadelphia Eagles, contributing to their loss of the Super Bowl championship game and subsequent years of underachievement. Of course there are exceptions, but they tend to prove the rule. For example, the Los Angeles Lakers won championships while the team's two stars, Shaquille

O'Neal and Kobe Bryant, disliked and socially avoided each other. But the coach, Phil Jackson, adept in Zen Buddhism, initially used the force of their personality conflicts to bind the team together to achieve a uniquely gritty *esprit de corps*. When Shaq and Kobe's animosity reached a level of intensity that the coach and his spiritual ministrations could no longer bind, the team began to lose its focus and suffered a decline in its play. Jackson rightly claimed that the team had lost its soul.[75] When members of the Budapest String Quartet came to dislike each other enough to avoid traveling together on concert tours, their music-making suffered an analogous decline in spirit, as others and I directly experienced with mounting disappointment.

The Limits on Socializing

I have given examples throughout our discussions of group members socializing together: going out to dinner, attending concerts and parties, visiting each other's homes. In the process, they have typically come to care about each other more than if their relationships had been strictly confined to official group meetings. Yet, as to be expected, sometimes the outside socializing has not clicked and, rather than increase feelings of closeness, has possibly diminished them, even to the point of animosity. But in a spiritual group animosities must not be allowed to become entrenched. If they cannot be resolved with dispatch, then some among those involved may have to be referred elsewhere. Otherwise the group cannot achieve its mission of promoting spiritual growth and achieving an encompassing group spirit.

From what has been implied, there are very good reasons that this emotionally intense type of therapy should not be casually undertaken: it may be dangerous not only to the participants but even to people in the outside world. The following vignette is a grim reminder of just how fraught the undertaking can become if it is not properly structured and attentively monitored.

Helene and Bernard

An attorney Bernard and a real estate developer Helene were referred to me by the same therapist several months apart. Both were depressed and doing poorly in their professions. Despite often losing money and being sued, Helene had completed several high-profile projects in the city, which, unknown to me, Bernard knew of and admired. Bernard had several times before started real estate partnerships but often failed to bring them to successful fruition. As I later found out, prior to therapy with me the two had been introduced and discussed doing a project together, but so far nothing had come of their discussions. Not knowing about their past association, I assigned them to the same group. My mistake, compounded by my not knowing their track records, soon became obvious.

Bernard and Helene gave a party at Bernard's house, and everyone who attended, with the exception of Bernard's wife, belonged to the therapeutic community. This included members of my other groups, who were marital partners of members of Bernard and Helene's group. Permission for such a party had been mentioned and at least tacitly given by the group, over which I had failed to exercise adequate oversight. Over drinks and hors d'oeuvres at the party, the main topics of conversations were idealized notions of my skills as a therapist and mischievous gossip about various members' personal lives. More alarming, there was much self-congratulatory talk of how special those in attendance were. The "have-nots," mainly spouses and parents, had the common distinction of not belonging to the therapeutic community. Even though many of them, as a matter of record, were seekers of psychological growth through therapy, they had "clearly" subscribed to an inferior brand of it, allegedly lacking the breadth and spirituality of the partygoers' path. Religious groups also came in for criticism because of their alleged formality and failure to promote emotional closeness among congregation members. Very little conversation was devoted to the members' common everyday interests, the usual content of healthy social interactions. The main common interest, their shared goal of psychological and spiritual maturation, was apparently mentioned in passing but not manifested to an appreciable degree.

With a growing sense of invulnerability after the party, Helene and Bernard went on to launch a large real estate development that within a few months failed and caused them both to be sued by the partners of the venture. They in turn threatened to sue me for fostering their unholy alliance, a suit that foundered on their past association. But there was enough blame to go around. My acceptance of multiple referrals from the same source, no matter how flattering and well intentioned, certainly should have set off alarm bells calling for a detailed assessment of the circumstances of the referrals.

This cautionary tale illustrates the real dangers of attempting to spiritualize outpatient groups by outside socializing without adequate rules and oversight. The most important rule broken here was the prohibition against financial dealings between the members, of equal importance to the rule against romantic and sexual relations. What is not so obvious and has not been discussed before is that despite an overall emphasis on outside socializing in spiritualizing a group, this should not often extend to large group socializing. The danger of outside meetings can be directly correlated with the size of the group. Groups of five tend to be more dangerous than threesomes, and threesomes, with their tendency toward triangulation, are greatly more dangerous than twosomes. By and large then, meetings on the outside should mostly be limited to pairs, and any larger grouping should for the most part be confined to the therapist's office under supervision. It would, of course, be unreasonable not to allow several group members to attend a party in which they constituted a minority of the whole and agreed not to discuss their joint therapy, a discussion that, in any case, would constitute a violation of confidentiality and privacy.

As mentioned previously, these proposed meetings of pairs—or occasionally, in special cases, of threes or fours—must have a rationale that secures the approval of the sponsoring group and its leaders. After these forays on the outside, the pair must report sources of comfort and discomfort and any occurrences of untoward events. Group discussions are then undertaken to correct problems and improve the learning potential of future ventures. Only with the acceptance of this kind of accountability can a group truly be said to sponsor the extra-group practices of members.

Needless to say, all these rules were broken by Helene and Bernard, mainly because the rules' absolute necessity was not fully appreciated by me and my co-therapist at the time. When this series of untoward events took place, I had not yet come to terms with how carefully the evaluation and monitoring processes had to be put in place before we allowed any outside get-togethers; nor was the need to restrict the process to pairs or very small subgroups of members understood. By the time the mistakes were recognized, the sled full of speculators was racing down a steep slope toward a stone wall. Despite all attempts to divert the impending collision, the time had passed for doing so. The unrealistic fantasies fueling this misadventure should have been stopped before their initial enactments.

Cult Formation

What we see in the experience with Helene and Bernard are the precursors of cult formation. We start with a social gathering driven by the unrealistic, neurotic needs of instigators, who proceed to idealize the abilities of a leader or leaders. The gathering is not bound by rules that dispel the tendency of groups to become a mob, with its characteristic psychology of maximizing the aggrandizement of an in-group and the minimization of an out-group, processes that easily lead to absolutist certainty about one's own abilities and beliefs and intolerance of that of others. Such intolerance, in a worshipful séance of leaders and entranced acolytes, typically overflows into a derogation of the families of origin and the social institutions of the recruited individuals, thereby releasing them from the restraints of the values and mores derived from their prior upbringing. At its worst, members of such a mob can financially, physically, and sexually abuse their followers, not stopping short of mass murder, as in the Jonestown tragedy of 1978 and the Stalin purges of the 1930 and 1940s, or on a lesser scale of evil, the mass financial ruin and economic recession starting in 2008 of subscribers to the risky schemes that had been misleadingly and greedily promoted by a maniacally interconnected group of subprime lenders.

The Madoff Ponzi scheme, in which Holocaust survivors and charities, among others, lost $60 billion of their savings, was the most salient example of a type of cultish economic behavior. Madoff created an exclusive club of celebrity clients and feeders of clients who were taken in by his unctuous warmth and apparent benevolence in giving the investors an apparent annual return of 10 percent on their investments. He apparently gave more to the feeder investment firms, who accepted management fees from clients without doing any management, just turning all the money over to Madoff because of his obvious superiority as an investor. In nineteenth-century psychiatry, Madoff and those who knowingly misled and grievously harmed their clients would have been given the diagnosis of moral insanity, which pretty well hits the nail on the head. More rational actors would appreciate not only the evil but the intrinsic self-destructiveness and Self-destructiveness of such a scheme, even involving the suicide of one of Madoff's sons. Nowadays schemers like Madoff and his associates are commonly given the diagnosis of antisocial personality disorder. Making such a prosaic diagnosis in this case misses the mark by a whole universe, a universe where good and evil are essential attributes. This would be like characterizing Hitler and Idi Amin's murderous schemes as manifestations of unresolved hostility.

Cults

There are few topics more fascinating to the social therapist than the powerful attraction of cults for alienated moderns. How pernicious one judges this attraction to be depends on which cultish organizations we are talking about: the Branch Davidians (Waco, 1993), Synanon "hair cutters," and Jonestown Kool-Aid drinkers on the one hand or the Moonies, Hare Krishnas, and Scientologists on the other. Since the former have tended to demand total subjugation of the individual will to the group will, in some cases leading to criminality and even mass suicide, we have little trouble judging them to be pernicious. But what about the more loosely organized and less obviously coercive quasi-religious groups such as the latter? For example, Scientology, like the Synanon-derived abusive behavior modification programs, promotes anti-scientific beliefs about medical care, resulting in poorly treated illnesses and needless morbidity and death. Proponents of Scientology, such as certain celebrity film actors, are notorious for their rants against the field of psychiatry even as they manifest alarming behavior on talk shows and elsewhere.

Irrational belief systems such as the Church of Synanon share with other cults the capacity to inspire destructive courses of action en masse. In one notorious case members put silenced rattlesnakes in the mailboxes of enemies. This is because the intensity of group loyalty inspired by these cults gives the leaders mind control over their adherents, often to a greater degree and to more nefarious purpose than is found in devotees to mainstream religions. But rather than weigh in more fully on the contentious issues of which specific groups qualify as benign or pernicious cults, I will leave it to authorities on cults to name names. For such an enterprise, how Wilhelm Reich's theory of character armor,[76] a major contribution to therapy practice, degenerated into the cultish Orgone Box therapy, is a prime candidate for discussion. Instead of taking on these broader cult effects, however, we will narrow our focus to trying to define the properties and attractions of therapeutic cults and the prospects for finding healthier alternatives.

Attractions and Dangers

Individuals who join cults tend to manifest certain characteristics, such as passive submissiveness to "magical" authority and depressive personalities that make them especially vulnerable to the cults' seductive claims of having final answers to the mysteries and perplexities of life. Their vulnerability becomes extreme when they suffer social isolation, cultural alienation, personal chaos, and loss of employment. Cults powerfully address the hunger, loneliness, and loss of self-esteem that accompany these circumstances. The comfort afforded by buying into the cult's ideology and membership and accepting its resources comes at the steep price of forfeiting individual freedom and responsibility.

In the aftermath of the several genocides and wholesale destruction of the wars of the twentieth century, the need for a rational belief system that promised to redeem the losses and dislocations went largely unmet. In many cases, the failure of mainstream religions to give answers contributed to their widespread loss of credibility. This left a spiritual vacuum that cults and extremist gangs have rushed in to fill. Moreover, in this time of rapid cultural change spawned by globalization and the information technology revolution, not only churches but also political causes and other traditional associations no longer capture the full attention of many who formerly turned to them for a sense of social connection. This is particularly true for legions of teenagers and young adults from broken homes and high-rise city dwellings who have drifted into deviant, destructive subcultures of drug-taking and gang warfare, in the absence of constructive alternatives.

So what is so dangerous about cults? Confining ourselves to those that promise therapy or healing, the dictionary definition of a therapeutic cult is "a system for the cure of disease based on the dogma, tenets, or principles set forth by its promulgators to the exclusion of scientific experiment or demonstration."[77] The danger derives from the nature of their dogma coupled with their mind control over acolytes. Cult leaders tend, by definition, to be dogmatic ideologues who have concocted doctrines and programs mainly out of personal neurotic and even psychotic needs rather than the transpersonal requirements of pragmatic benefits and social justice. Driven by deep-seated personal inadequacies, cult followers betray an excessive devotion to such leaders and their ideas. Those who study cults discover that this leader-worship, even with its fascistic, grandiose narcissism, would not be so dangerous were it not for two additionally malignant factors: one, that it often demands of its adherents, in a brainwashing mode, the renunciation of family, friends, and the values of the surrounding society—which might be justifiable in a vicious police state but only serves to tear the social fabric of a reasonably benign, already chaotic democracy; and two, the dangerous cult is a closed society, virtually prohibiting its members from leaving once they have been recruited, sometimes prompting concerned family members to hire abductors and deprogrammers to get their loved ones back. With their "no way out" aspect coupled with persistent indoctrination, the net result can be an annihilation of the individual personalities of converts. Cult followers, now untied from their moorings to time-honored obligations and morals, have renounced their individual critical will in submission to the will of the cult leadership. All the ingredients are now in place for the lowest common denominator of the group to take over and induce the mass psychotic behavior described by LeBon in the French Revolution and witnessed in every age since—from Salem to the Holocaust to radical Islamism.

The recommended alternative is a therapeutic group that meets the needs that cults address while leaving the members their freedom and autonomy. Such groups are then ready to be spiritualized—that is, to create a group spirit exemplifying the highest spiritual values derived from group consciousness. This process must be carried out in a carefully thought-out, principled fashion for the requisite emotional attraction and interpersonal bonding to be achieved on safe terms. Yet those who hope to run a spiritual therapeutic program according to sound principles always have to be mindful of the intensely connected group's potential for sliding into behavior that is cult-like: anti-society, anti-family, absolutist, exclusionary, and exploitative, to name just a few of the cult's most hazardous attributes. What I want to discuss finally and more fully are the philosophy and safeguards that must be put in place to thwart such a development.

The Treatment Philosophy

In our prior discussions of the treatment philosophy of the outpatient milieu approach, we have emphasized the multidimensional application of all recognized techniques of intervention, covering the spectrum of the biological, psychosocial, and spiritual realms. In an effort to reduce symptoms and promote psychological and moral growth, we have advocated an activist utilization of the latest knowledge about pharmacology; psychodynamic, cognitive, and behavioral psychology; applied sociology and anthropology; and the techniques of enhanced awareness in promoting moral and spiritual development. Although we have discussed the advisability, as a practical matter, of avoiding sectarian commitments in promoting this multidimensional agenda, we have not so far stressed the necessity of holding firm to this stance in avoiding cultish degeneration.

What this means is that we cannot afford to fall into either/or thinking about causes or clinical practices when we address psychiatric disorder. No symptom or syndrome is, with respect to etiology, all biologically or all psychologically or all spiritually determined. A patient's depression is not the result of a chemical imbalance alone. Some aspects of the depressed person's feelings and behavior are also the product of past learning and present emotional conflicts. Other aspects are the product of spiritual deficits: a lack of faith in oneself and the possibility of social progress; a lack of a belief system that supports creative and healing ideals; a failure of resolve to take action against all negative feelings and states of being, to turn them into positives. These factors always act concurrently to produce symptomatic behaviors, even though we may choose to treat them by serially deploying biological, psychosocial, and spiritual remedies.

Similarly, from the psychological perspective, emotional problems are not the result of either Freudian psychodynamic or Beckian cognitive-behavioral factors; both perspectives offer useful insights and methods of intervention. And spiritual influences do not come wrapped in exclusively Jungian or Rankian or Christian or Judaic forms. Each form, each perspective, may have something to offer. Yet the biggest mistake of all, in the service of a misguided distaste for the medical model, is to exclude biological factors from the account of etiology and consequently resort to tortuously extended psychological explanations that preclude the prescribing of medication while justifying ever more intrusive behavior modification programs. These latter programs have sounded the death knell on Synanon-derived approaches, like some of the wilderness programs or other harsh confrontational methods that feel justified in exposing patients to verbal and even physical abuse, instead of, God forbid, having the patients swallow an unkosher pill or two.

Cults thrive on absolutist and fundamentalist thinking. "We are the way. We have the answer. We are right; the others are wrong and have to pay the price." This is a grandiose paranoid stance that depends on and feeds divisiveness. In contrast, the very essence of spirituality is an all-embracing inclusiveness. Moreover, spirituality embraces the positive over the negative, trying to see the good in order to maximize it and concentrating on the bad only to transform it, not to relish its blamefulness. On the one hand cults fabricate a paranoid pseudo-community; on the other, spiritual groups create a real community of tolerant and inclusive healers and creators. Just as the paranoid person is the epitome of the anti-spiritual individual, so the cult is the epitome of the pseudo-spiritual group.

The Rules of the Spiritual Group

In addition to screening out patients with bad character and malignant track records, the outpatient therapeutic community must have strict rules about outside socializing and about behavior toward the leader, members, and members' friends and family. Scrupulousness in these matters is essential to avoiding mob rule and cultish behavior. Let me reiterate some of the obvious principles.

1. All socializing outside the group has to be approved by the members for specific therapeutic purposes, and the course of these outside contacts must be fully reported to the group for processing. This socializing must be confined to very small subgroups, preferably pairs, to avert the emergence of cultish ingroupness.
2. No sexual or romantic involvement between members is allowed. If romances develop, one or both parties should be discharged from the parent group, although they may continue in separate groups. Each separate group is a symbolic immediate family, and family rules governing incest and prerogatives apply.
3. No financial dealings between members are allowed. Any help rendered, such as a lawyer or doctor member giving other members professional direction, must follow the paradigm of informal family help. They must be acts of friendship, in which money does not change hands.
4. Go Dutch. All bills, such as for meals or entertainment, are to be split equally or alternately.
5. There should be no parties in which milieu members outnumber "outsiders" and in which the program, the members, or the leader are topics of conversation.
6. Family, friends, and the larger society are not to be disparaged. If

a member is suffering at the hands of any of these, the focus has to be on the member's coping strategies, not on the moral valence of the apparent offenders. In particular, spouses of members are rarely to be explicitly criticized, nor should judgments be made about the advisability of terminating a marriage except in cases of severe, unremitting abuse.

7. Patients must not be dissuaded, much less forbidden, from leaving the spiritual community. The exercise of free will, encouraged by an open-door policy, is essential to fostering the spirituality of free men and women, whose autonomy must never be compromised by a fundamentalist "we know what's good for you" notion of truth, unless mental incompetence is manifest.

Group members who do not follow these rules, even though they agreed to do so, are the source of the main problems that afflict the group milieu. In one sense, this inability to observe legitimate rules is the behavioral essence of what we mean by flawed or bad character. Its spiritual essence is a lack of effective moral conscience. We must define these terms so that we can recognize greater and lesser degrees of character and character disorder, the subject of the next chapter.

Chapter 8
CHARACTER DEVELOPMENT

Summary. Since character and character strength are operational embodiments of the individual's value system, character determines to a significant degree the individual's destiny. By the same token, character fortifies will, particularly self-discipline and active striving. In addition to corralling internal saboteurs, will-strengthened character is essential to mitigating the common tendencies toward obesity, promiscuity, passivity, arrogance, envy, and rage, the so-called deadly sins. Daily rituals are important tools of combat. The most basic ritual is an exercise program that is used to anchor the will. To this anchor other routines are tied, to institute a range of curbings and strivings in the service of spiritual values. These rituals constitute gymnastics of both the body and the soul. Through the practice of the gymnastics, character is forged in the crucible of sweat and tears, pain and defeat, joy and fulfillment. Building character to further the welfare of both the individual self and the common Self, our collective being, propels us down the road to living a spiritual life.

Character is destiny, or simply put, what we are made of greatly determines what becomes of us. Character is defined as "a composite of good moral qualities typically of moral excellence and firmness blended with resolution, self-discipline, high ethics, force, and judgment."[78] Since character includes our guiding values as well as our power and judgment to realize them, it writes the plotline of our life story, with its successes and failures, its loyalties and betrayals. It determines how we react to the most important crises of our lives. Do we stand firm when greed or fear threatens to overwhelm our sense of right? Do we crumble when we lose a job or a loved one? Or do we grieve and then consolidate our resources to become stronger and more determined? Success, no less than loss, is also a great test of character. Some respond to high achievement with a heightened sense of gratitude and responsibility, whereas others fall victim to arrogance and an overweening sense of entitlement.

Such far-reaching claims about the consequences of character make sense only if we recognize how inextricably it is bound up with spiritual values. Character, as defined, is essentially a moral attribute that connotes steadfastness, determination, and integrity. People with strong character do not "hit-and-run" but rather "stick and stand." They do not abandon loved ones or causes because they are no longer pretty or popular. They do not disaffiliate from a persecuted minority to avoid public opprobrium and unfair treatment. Nor do they sell out to the highest bidder, unless the bid is for the highest good. In contrast, saying that people have bad or flawed character means that they are fickle and shallow; they cannot be relied on to come through in the clutch. And they are capable of betraying friends and family for personal gain or in fealty to a cause or belief system whose intemperate embrace may have more to do with psychological need than with intellectual merit. Because character is fundamentally about loyalty and personal integrity, it is the most basic spiritual quality of the individual.

My first conscious encounter with strong character came in childhood; it was an occurrence that my family always reminiscences about at our reunions. My grandmother Frieda, who lived with us in the rural South, came from Eastern Europe. She taught our African American cook Lula, who worked for us for more than a quarter-century, how to make many traditional Jewish dishes. She also schooled her in some of the Jewish dietary laws, which were not easy to observe in our small town in the white-bread, Bible Belt South. But Lula, welcoming the challenge, did more than anyone could rightfully expect. Grandma Frieda died early in 1942, which Lula took very hard. When Passover came in springtime, Mother told her we weren't going to change our everyday dishes for the special Passover dishes this year. Lula was outraged and declared vehemently, "Mrs. Abroms, you do that, and I quit." She meant it. We changed the dishes that year and every Passover as long as Lula lived. Because of her, the family held on to part of its cultural heritage, strengthening its overall sense of ethnic identity. And we continue to carry Lula in our hearts. One of the ways my family tries to repay our debt to Lula is to support the integration of African Americans into American society and to promote their financial and cultural well-being. We take pride in having a well-qualified African American president, even when we disagree with his politics. In general, abandoning one's support of a persecuted minority, no less than abandoning one's membership in it, tends to speak poorly of one's character. Of course, there are exceptions, especially when survival is threatened, and disloyalty is the only viable alternative.

Lula was loyal to the memory of my grandmother Frieda and what she stood for. Since my mother worked, Frieda was Lula's main teacher and mentor. Lula in turn was a second mother to everyone in the family. I spent most of my childhood under her feet in the kitchen, sampling her unique mix of the cuisines of the Deep South and the Eastern European shtetl. Black-eyed peas, fried chicken, grits, *tsimmes*, *grebenes*, and *kugel* make for an unforgettably exotic cuisine that is not easy to find in the restaurants of our time, even those that lay claim to high fusion.

The quality of our gratitude to the memory of our teachers and loved ones and our responses to violations of our loyalties, to intimidation, to devastating loss, and to being given unfair advantages or taken advantage of—all these constitute holograms of our moral fiber, our character. In the next chapter, we will examine the role of empathy, another major precondition of developing a spiritual life.

Character and Character Disorders

In the rush to moral neutrality, "character" and "character disorder" are terms that have been excised from psychiatric diagnostic manuals because they are so obviously value-laden. To say that people are lacking in character or have character flaws is to say that they are one or more of the following: unreliable, weak, corruptible, dishonest, manipulative, shallow, or disloyal. To say that they have character disorders is to further specify that they manifest these bad qualities in characteristic patterns of abuse, exploitation, and betrayal. I am not recommending that these terms be reintroduced into the personality disorder section of the *Diagnostic and Statistical Manual*, the empirical rule book governing the scientific discourse of psychiatric disorders, but rather am suggesting that we assign them to the realm of the spiritual discourse on these disorders, where they are looked upon as moral failings in need of moral treatment. As I have defined it, moral treatment involves an infusion of spirit, an infusion of tough and tender love and will by respected teachers, who thereby qualify as mentors.

To say that someone has character, rather than a lack of it, is to say that he or she is steadfast, resolute, and honest, that the individual's commitment can be counted on, and that the individual can be trusted to remain loyal—so long as his or her trust has not been betrayed. Persons of character are also understood to have high degrees of genuineness and authenticity; that is, they are true to themselves. In chapter 1, I suggested that everyone has a core being and that discovering and developing it is the essence of spiritual growth and the source of one's uniqueness as a human being. Character as affirmed authenticity, as being true to one's core self, is what guides us to believe in, stand for, and live by principles that grow out of our true being.

Not everyone is comfortable talking about human beings in such morally judgmental terms. Pointing to character flaws seems to render rigid verdicts about incorrigible human weakness, as if to say that some are morally strong, and others are frail, with no way out for the weaklings. Obviously, spiritual therapists do not see the matter in this way. As Maimonides maintained, we can develop our character by repeated acts of will, in the service of becoming better people, of becoming ever closer to our authentic selves and to closing the gap between self and Self. In doing so, we come to stand steadfastly for the right values and to live righteously. I think this will become clear if we look at the kinds of situations that call for strength of character and that, painfully and often, expose weaknesses in our own character and behavior. But first we must own up to the elusiveness of character assessment.

Uncertainties about Character Assessment

Having made categorical statements about character, we must step back and acknowledge that the subject has a large measure of ambiguity. Essential to the thrust of this book, the possibility surely exists that individuals can undergo psychological and spiritual growth in character strength, that life experiences can serve as crucibles for purifying and hardening character. And we must not forget that we may misjudge people because we are lacking in important knowledge about them.

For example, many years ago during my stint in the Air Force, my wife and I became friendly with another couple but gradually grew exasperated with their behavior. She appeared to be a spoiled brat, always asking him to fetch things or begging out of swimming or sightseeing ventures on account of the heat or the humidity. She lay around fanning herself and expecting to be catered to, an attitude incongruous with the heightened-alert status of a Strategic Air Command base during the Cold War. Writing her off as a princess indulged by a henpecked husband, we drew apart.

Bad characters? Not so fast. As it turned out, our assessment was flawed. Some years later we discovered that the wife had died on the operating table during an effort to repair a congenital heart defect that was causing congestive heart failure. What we had witnessed years before was the couple's valiant efforts to hide her compromised cardiopulmonary function. That she accompanied her husband on this military assignment in an area remote from expert cardiac care, and took pains not to be pitied for her disability, required courage and effort on both their parts. One may question their judgment and extreme pride in not sharing the particulars of her condition, but we can hardly absolve ourselves from the rush to harsh judgment, in total ignorance of the true situation.

Character comes in many shades and is not always evident from a casual observation of behavior. What may first appear to be a hologram or microcosm of a person's basic character may later prove to be a transient distortion. And even if it is not, we cannot assume that a character weakness is refractory to repair, given enough dedication and ingenuity. We derive hope and inspiration from those rare individuals who have abandoned a life of addiction and promiscuity to become contributing members of society. Despite our tendency to sentence people to unpardonable verdicts, we must exercise great caution in making these assessments of moral value. Judgments of character must always be tempered, held as provisional hypotheses, subject to change with greater knowledge and effort. Although it is uncommon, even habitual criminals can sometimes go straight and make a contribution to society. The rarity of the phenomenon has partly to do with the difficulty of reining in a split-off, tension-reducing, law-breaking internal saboteur, whose manifestations we have discussed previously. One may also assume that genetics play a significant role in criminal behavior, although the evidence remains incomplete.

Predictive Value of Character Assessment

· Despite exceptions, the concept of character remains useful because it points to a relatively stable aspect of an individual's personality. Cautiously considered, it can have predictive value, for if we can cogently assess character structure, we can more accurately foresee the reliability of individuals in times of adversity and determine how much potential they have for growth and repair. As the following vignette makes clear, these predictions are sometimes thrown off by a lack of the material resources necessary for patients to make good on their intentions.

Sam, a hospital technician from a family of petty criminals, married Doris, a physician from a professional family. She subsidized his education and bore him a child. In the mode of "no good deed goes unpunished,"

Sam repaid her by stealing the password and substantial funds from her savings account. Sam's theft of his wife Doris's savings clearly illustrates the workings of a severe character defect, characterized by law-breaking hostile ingratitude and what psychodynamic theorists might label as superego lacunae, the consequence of being raised by criminals. The case also raises some of the complex issues of assessing the potential for remediation. The betrayal involved in stealing from a wife who was paying for his schooling and therapy was so appalling that many of Doris's friends begged her to kick Sam out immediately. But since he expressed genuine remorse and vowed to work hard to pay off his debt, she judged that he was not a true psychopath and that he was sincere in his resolve to rebalance his moral ledger. In consequence, Doris delayed giving Sam the boot, while insisting that he scrupulously pay off his debt and assume his current responsibilities as husband and father.

He made a game effort to do so: he was mostly reliable in caring for their infant son and did the chores he was supposed to perform. But he couldn't earn enough money to make a dent in his debt, even after he gave up college and therapy. Over time Doris realized that despite Sam's sincere efforts, she could not recover her love and trust. In asking him to move out, she realized that divorce was inevitable. Sam had demonstrated that he did not have the character structure of a conscienceless psychopath by the quality of his remorse and his partially realized intentions of acting responsibly, but as with many who try to go straight, he did not have the human capital to completely control his impulses and to learn a discipline that would earn him a good living. His plan to become an X-ray technician fell through when he failed to show up regularly for classes. He seemed destined to earn the pay of a low-level technician.

Despite such disappointments, it is important for therapists to make an all-out effort in these cases because patients sometimes surprise us with the magnitude of their changes. A case in point is the example of the patient mentioned in an earlier chapter who overcame sexual abuse and many years of addiction and failed marriages to become abstinent, earn a business degree, and form a stable family. At the very least, making the effort helps develop a more realistic idea of who will respond to our help and how much we can expect from them and ourselves given the mental, physical, and material resources available.

Refusing to Be Compromised

Sometimes we are put in situations that cast doubt on our integrity through no fault of our own. Someone has quoted us falsely, attributed bad motives to innocent behavior, or betrayed our confidential advice. Our reputation can also suffer from the company we keep. How we respond to such situations both tests and defines our character. Even though it is not always wise to respond to allegations of impropriety, for fear of dignifying them, there are still many times when we must actively resist efforts to compromise our good name. How best to do it can present a terrible dilemma.

For example, Albert was very proud to be marrying Angela. Not only was she lovely, but her family was also distinguished, in contrast to his own. A dark secret for Albert was that his father had been indicted for possible embezzlement years earlier. All went well until after the wedding reception, when Angela's father went to pay the band. The $3,000 in cash he had placed in his coat pocket was missing! Had he forgotten to transfer the money to his pocket?

Fast-forward to several days later when the family was gathered to review the videotapes of the wedding affair. Lo and behold, Albert's father had been captured apparently reaching into the inner pocket of Angela's father's jacket, draped over the back of a chair. In the stink that followed, Albert's father vehemently denied that he had taken anything, claiming that he was only straightening the jacket to keep it from falling off the chair. Albert loyally defended his father. Angela was now gagging on the bitter dregs of what had so recently been a delicious wedding wine. Not surprisingly, the marriage was already doomed.

Does this episode tell us anything about Albert's character? We are not concerned here with his father, whose deficits apparently went beyond character flaws into the realm of outright criminality. How might Albert have handled the episode to better effect? It is usually an admirable trait to stand by your own family in squabbles with outsiders. And certainly the evidence against his father was, although strong, inconclusive. Yet there was, at the very least, an appearance of impropriety, and Albert's own honor, as well as that of his family, was at stake. Should he not have done something more than merely defend his father against the allegation of theft? Was there any way to do this without betraying his family? One thing he might have done was insist on reimbursing his father-in-law for the money lost and show allegiance to his wife and new in-laws by restricting his own family's access to them, leaving aside the question of his father's guilt. Such a course of action at least would have kept open the possibility of restoring trust in the integrity of the marriage. No doubt, there were other possibilities. But merely defending his father in this situation did not testify to good character. It did not demonstrate a strong resolve to do whatever was necessary to salvage his marital covenant by showing good faith to his new family.

There is no greater test of character than being faced with the dishonesty of parents or esteemed mentors. Loyalty assuredly dictates that they should be given the benefit of the doubt, but the price may be the destruction of one's own credibility and integrity. Certainly we are enjoined to honor our parents and to be thankful for all they have done for us: bringing us into the world and taking care of us and supporting our education. Yet to build our own character, the time may come when we must separate ourselves from their behavior and values, and this becomes particularly evident when our welfare, not just our good name, is jeopardized.

The Cheater

Freddy was known to be a cheater by his tennis partners, as I found out by happenstance from an acquaintance who was one of these partners. These old friends said he was "twisted" but could not help himself. In loyalty to their childhood friendship, they kept him in the game, overruling his line calls as needed. Some time back, he had temporarily lost his medical license for insurance fraud. Once he was again in good standing, he took his physician son Michael into his practice as full partner. After a few years the opportunity arose to sell the practice to a hospital for a large sum. But when Freddy divided up the proceeds, Michael complained bitterly that he was not getting his fair share. Freddy was adamant that his apportionment was right, and he even enlisted Michael's mother to his side. In their rage and revulsion at this seeming betrayal, Michael and his wife decided that they could no longer socialize with his father and mother, although they decided against a lawsuit. Michael's mother, devastated at not being able to see her grandchildren, became severely depressed. She was referred to me for treatment. In recognizing the family name, I connected the story she told me to the old story of Freddy's cheating at tennis. Of course, I was in no position to use this information other than to suggest the possibility of a miscalculation in the disbursement of funds, which she firmly and immediately dismissed.

In consideration of his mother's depression Michael relented to the extent of allowing the grandparents a weekly supervised visit with the grandchildren. Freddy and his wife could never bring themselves to admit that perhaps a mistake had been made or that some concessions should be offered.

In the absence of further knowledge, it would appear that Michael and his wife showed considerable strength of character in how they dealt with this situation. They firmly separated themselves from Freddy's pattern of dishonesty by maintaining a stance of disapproval and social distance. Yet they honored their family bond by preserving the relationship between grandparents and grandchildren and refusing to take legal action against Michael's father Freddy.

Questions remain as to whether or not Michael should have forgiven his parents or should have given them the benefit of the doubt. Even though this might be a reasonable position, insisting on it from the outset moves us toward the suspect "negotiated human relations" view of the world, where all conflicts can be resolved by communication and compromise. This is a worldview in which there is little room for old-fashioned absolutes such as character and moral truth. Although it is possible that Michael was at fault or at least was unforgiving, it is more likely that, having worked closely with his father in their medical practice and in their family life together, he had come to know all too well what Freddy's tennis partners had discovered: that he was a cheater. But until this episode, Michael had not believed his father would cheat his own son. He did not realize that there was such a thing as moral insanity, which honors no sacred bonds and therefore yields an "equal opportunity" cheater. But he did recognize that his own character development required that he hold firm against his father's self-serving account of reality. A measure of forgiveness might come later, after he secured his own immunity from the damaging effects of being raised by parents who were so deeply flawed.

Accepting Responsibility

"We were just obeying orders." When German and Serbian soldiers were accused of genocide during a century-long nightmare of mass murders and ethnic cleansing, atrocities that continue to this very day in Africa and the Middle East, they often resorted to this evasion of responsibility, vehemently so once their parts in the massacres could no longer be denied. They were not at fault, so they alleged, because they had been ordered to commit murder by others whom they were forced to obey.

Fortunately, this rationalization has forever been discredited by the Adolph Eichmanns of the world. No matter who gave the orders, we cannot be absolved of personal responsibility for taking the lives of innocent human beings who are no threat to our own. Nor should we get away with claiming we were only cogs in the transportation machine that conveyed prisoners to the gas chambers. Driving the "go to" car is no better than driving the getaway car. Yet these "superior orders" and "cog in the machine" defenses have remained the benchmarks, the extreme cases, against which all failures to take personal responsibility are measured and put into perspective. Every day we see large and small versions of passing the buck, claiming bad luck, blaming the envied, or invoking conspiracy, all in an effort to deny our own responsibility for what we have done to ourselves or others. To do otherwise, to stand up and come clean about our complicity in the failures that are always mixed in with our successes, takes more strength of character than most of us possess. It is heartening to witness those rare occasions when someone owns squarely up to what he or she has done and resolves to do better.

Ned the Carpenter

Ned, a carpenter, allowed his helper son Mark to take a recreational day off even though he needed him on a building job. On this fateful day, Mark played with a friend at an abandoned building site, using a hanging cable to swing from girder to girder. When the cable snapped, Mark fell and banged his head, dying later from a brain hemorrhage. In therapy, Ned faced up to his responsibility: he should have insisted that Mark come to work because he needed his help and because he needed to stop being an indulgent father, which he had increasingly become in battling his divorced wife for their children's favor.

I was astonished that rather than feeling more devastated by owning up, Ned was rescued from bottomless guilt. His grief was cut down to manageable size because he recognized that he could do something about the laxness that had been a contributing factor to Mark's death. Soon afterward, his daughter asked him for financial help in buying a car. But since Mark's death, she had had a series of auto accidents that indicated poor attention, if not outright self-destructiveness. With the support of his group, Ned refused to finance the car until his daughter demonstrated greater competence as a driver. When instead she persuaded her mother to buy the car for her, Ned was urged by his group to write his ex-wife a letter, with a copy to their daughter, avowing that if anything happened to her or anyone else as a result of her careless driving, he would hold his ex-wife personally responsible. The daughter became a much more careful driver after that. Ned felt that the group helped him to stand up to his ex-wife and daughter for the good of everyone.

By this act of tough love, Ned took a stand against the kind of permissiveness that had contributed to the death of his son. In doing so, he atoned for his past laxness and strengthened his character. He demonstrated that strength in a way that may have impeded his daughter's throwing away her life too. In taking some responsibility for his son's demise, a courageous act, and standing firm against his daughter's destructiveness, he partially redeemed himself and became a stronger person, as evidenced later on by a greater ability to stand his ground in other parts of his life. The major role Ned's group played in this outcome, giving him the support he needed to assert himself, cannot be overemphasized.

Ned's actions serve as an example of taking a characterful stand. If only we could always admit when we have given bad advice or misdiagnosed a patient or failed to repay debts of gratitude. Instead we often blame the economy or the patient's poor communication or a friend's minor slights to justify our negligence or lack of generosity. Each time, we not only betray our weakness of character but also miss the opportunity to strengthen it.

Realizing Potential

The veneer of relativity that always covers such seeming absolutes as good character and moral worth is at no time more evident than when we try to measure them. In one sense, of course, we are all equally worthy in that each of us is a manifestation of the life force, of the animating Spirit behind the sensory world. But in another sense, such moral leveling offends our sense of justice. Although all are self-evidently born equal, surely some contribute more and lead more exemplary lives than others. How can a Hitler or a Stalin be mentioned in the same breath as an Abraham Lincoln or a Martin Luther King Jr.? What is true about the latter two is that each man overcame enormous obstacles to better the lives of his people. And what is tragically true of the former two is that they betrayed their endowment of leadership genius to tear rather than repair the fabric of the world.

But what do such extreme examples tell us about the character and moral worth of more ordinary people like ourselves, who are paragons neither of good nor of evil but who nevertheless try to lead good lives? They tell us that we should be judged not only by how well we do in an absolute sense but also by how well we do with the hand we have been dealt—in other words, how well we realize out potential, however great or small it is. Our character is measured by how close we come to doing our best with our endowment. By this standard, Franklin D. Roosevelt's success in overcoming the limitations of his polio-crippled body and his insular patrician upbringing to lead the United States out of economic depression, to provide a safety net for the poor, and to spearhead the war effort against a grave threat to Western democracy is a supreme example of character as realized potential despite elitist upbringing and severe physical disability. Perhaps more impressive was Dr. King's ability to overcome his racial disenfranchisement to lead his people and a whole nation toward the promised land of racial tolerance. The true character of each man can be fully appreciated only by taking account of what each overcame to realize his potential for doing the good, not just the absolute value of the good itself.

For us ordinary citizens who do not author world-shaking events or artistic works of genius, this dimension of our character is measured by the less august achievements of physical and mental development. Have we done our best to keep our bodies in shape through regular exercise and healthy diet, or have we succumbed to the epidemics of overeating and passive watching that tend to afflict members of affluent societies? Have we honed our intellectual and artistic skills to the fullest by informing ourselves about the political, economic, scientific, and cultural developments of our world? Are we assiduous in deepening our talents as artists, teachers, inventors, and healers? The more we pursue excellence in these skills, the stronger our character becomes. Failing to develop our endowment to the fullest, barring tragic circumstances outside our control, diminishes our character strength.

Of course, this is a difficult subject because we rarely know how prohibitive a person's circumstances are. We do not really know why Orson Welles and Marlon Brando did not fully deliver on their early promise. That both became extremely obese and that they did not maintain the levels of excellence demonstrated in their early work are generally agreed-upon observations. The same might be said of the Viennese composer Erich Korngold, who peaked in his early twenties as a prodigy as gifted as Mozart but ended up living the good life in Hollywood, while writing scores for Errol Flynn movies. In his case we do know some of the impactful adverse circumstances that may have altered his life course: he lost his homeland, his status, and his cultural support because of the Nazi occupation of Austria and the ban on Jewish art and music, soon to develop into genocide. (In Korngold's defense, he once again wrote great works after the Nazis were vanquished, just a few years before his death). Such incalculable losses are not often conducive to progress in artistic or spiritual development, despite Nietzsche's claim that the pain and losses that do not kill us only make us stronger. If only our character and resilience were always strong enough to make this wish come true.

The Deadly Sins

The most basic issue in individual character strength is self-discipline. Its absence has been defined by ancient scholars in their list of the seven deadly sins: arrogance (pride), envy, gluttony, greed, lust, rage, and sloth. Habitual excess in any of these personality traits is what we fundamentally mean by the lack of self-control that lies at the heart of weak or flawed character. Losing control—of appetites (greed, gluttony), of drives (lust, rage), and of overweening attitudes (arrogance, envy)—characterizes the first six sins. The seventh, sloth, is the catch-all for the various manifestations of passive-dependency and regression. Curbing and striving are the counterforces that must be applied to each of these tendencies. Success is measured in terms of the ability to maintain initiative, self-discipline, moderation, and balance—yet another list of the defining qualities of a healthy character.

1. Loss of Control of Appetites

Greed. Health and love are probably the only qualities we cannot have too much of. Material possessions head the list of what can become excessive and do fatal damage to the spiritual life. Greed is the driving appetite that cannot get enough of these possessions, the most corrupting of which are money, property, and dominating power. In a recent presidential election, one of the candidates owned so many homes that he somehow could not remember their number. His lack of candor spoke volumes about his guilty conscience and his poorly hidden greed for money and power.

As another example, Mr. Davidson, who started out as a small businessman, cornered the market on a product that made him a billionaire. But instead of using his wealth to support the arts and sciences or social causes, he used the bulk of it to buy large estates in the Hamptons, Palm Beach, and Santa Barbara and a private jet to ferry his celebrity friends to extravagant carnival weekends at these various sites. His garage in the Hamptons housed no fewer than fifteen antique and late-model European luxury cars. Mrs. Davidson compulsively shopped and accumulated closets full of expensive shoes, dresses, and furs. The Davidsons demanded of their employees and guests such deference and unqualified praise that after one of my patients took issue with Mr. Davidson for a disparaging remark about a mutual acquaintance's appearance, she and her husband were never invited on these weekend junkets again. Prior to that time they had regarded the Davidsons, who were godparents to their children and frequent guests in their home, as close friends of many years. Only gradually did my patient come to terms with the corrupting power of sudden wealth and greed on even "close friends."

Gluttony. Overeating has reached epidemic proportions in Western society, with a large percentage of the population qualifying as overweight. What is truly startling is that children are among the most afflicted. Even before we get to the distortions of character involved here, this is a public health crisis because the obese have a heightened vulnerability to a whole range of diseases, particularly cardiovascular and orthopedic conditions and metabolic conditions such as diabetes. Although the dangers of being overweight are sometimes exaggerated by the media, public health officials cringe to see American families consuming platters of pizza, cheeseburgers, and French fries, all washed down by sugar-rich drinks. Fortunately, cigarette smoking has been curbed, the connection with lung cancer having struck home for most Americans. But the dangers of overeating are only beginning to raise a similar alarm.

Beyond the physical health consequences, overindulgence in food and drink has dire consequences for character strength. By definition it is a prime indication of lack of willpower. To be able to say no to one's primitive appetites in favor of a higher good such as health is what we mean by willpower. Hunger for food is, of course, the most difficult of all appetites to curb, for our very life depends on its timely satisfaction. And the difficulty of the task explains why a prolonged hunger strike by the likes of a Gandhi can cause an empire to crumble. Perhaps if the Palestinians had declared hunger strikes instead of suicidal bombing strikes against Israeli occupation, they might have their own independent country by now. By such self-deprivation, a person or group demonstrates not only strength of will but also steadfastness of purpose and the very highest moral determination—in other words, superior character. There is every reason to believe that the eclipse of the British Empire was significantly abetted by such displays of superior moral strength on the part of colonial subjects. Many of the same points apply to curbing sexual and aggressive impulses, although these impulses are less immediately life-threatening and therefore carry less moral weight, both figuratively and literally. Needless to say, losing control of this self-denial process, as in anorexia or total pacifism, crosses over the line, sometimes a fine line, from character strength into pathology.

2. Loss of Control of Drives

Lust. It lubricates the axis on which the world spins. It throws our world out of orbit when lust crosses the border from passion to promiscuity, from desire to addiction. An indiscriminate expression of sexual passion—that is, doing it casually, addictively, or exploitatively with anyone who triggers arousal—debases the currency of both sex and love, for making love is not meant to be casual, not meant to be an entertainment or a plaything of the idle. Although the primitively sexual may experience lovemaking as little different from the tension relief afforded by other biological discharges, to richer souls the act offers the promise of engendering feelings of union and spiritual rapture, preparatory to the greatest creative act to which human beings are capable: giving birth to another being with a soul. An activity designed for the purpose of creating another person who also can grow up to be a spiritual being, jointly loved by his or her creators, is cheapened by putting it to any more casual use. Lovemaking ought to hold out the possibility of giving birth to a spiritual offspring, if not a real child then a symbolic one in the form of a valuable work (moral, aesthetic, or social) jointly authored out of mutual love overflowing into love for all. Otherwise, our betrayal of lovemaking's potential will culminate in postcoital blues, the sense, as clairvoyant schizophrenics sometimes tell us, of having wasted our vital essence.

But repeatedly making love to the wrong person, or in the wrong place, or at the wrong time, can do more damage than causing the blues. Lust can be so strong that good judgment and respect for the integrity of people and places are thrown out the window. The cost can be serious damage to a spouse or child, a family or organization, or even a cause. Businesses have imploded when managers have had illicit affairs with employees; the loss of trust and fear of favoritism are all-too-real threats to those who cannot escape the wanton evidence of these dalliances. Families break up when lust-driven pseudo-love bursts the bounds of privacy and discretion. Even if a case can be made for the place of casual sex between consenting adults, not everyone ends up feeling casual about the encounter, no matter what was said in the urgency of the moment. Lost mothers, lost fathers, lost children, and lost countries may be occasioned by the tearing apart after such tender intimacies, and the slide into a sense of betrayal ignites a fury almost as destructive as a suicide bomber at a family celebration.

Rage. The first overripe fruits of the psychotherapy revolution were unbridled expressions of rage toward parents and authorities, who were accused, often rightly so, of neglect and abuse. It took the better part of the last century for therapists and patients to come to their senses and realize that primal raging is simply bad behavior and rarely changes anything for the better—often, in fact, breaking apart already fragile bonds. Understand, I am not knocking appropriate expressions of anger, dissatisfaction, and competitive aggression. Rather, the culprit is unmodulated, destructive fury, a fury that places the blame for suffering totally on others, without respect for persons, places, and past debts and certainly without awareness that we all, to some extent, bring about what seems to be happening to us.

When stopped, the rageful always claim that they were just expressing their feelings. "You mean you want to deprive me of my right to express my feelings?" Actually, no, just your right to express them any way you like, without any sense of respect for others or doubt about your own perceptions or responsibilities. We see time and again how ballplayers lose their cool and attack referees, opponents, and even fans, in the process losing a game or even a whole season and certainly the credibility and respect earned by strong character. This is a microcosm of the larger world of human affairs, whether such things play out in the family, the school, the boardroom, the halls of international diplomacy, or when all reason is abandoned, the corpse-covered battlefield. We count on the strong character of leaders to rein in their own rage and their people's rage to avert the nuclear option.

In an academic department at a Midwestern university, faculty meetings often were disrupted by angry disputes over ideology and finances. A professor with no official position in the hierarchy of the department never took part in these disputes, confining his sparse remarks to clarification of factual details, although his own position was no secret. At the end of each of these melees, he would summarize the sense of the meeting, as if it were a Quaker gathering, and his summation was usually accepted as the final say. As to the source of his power, the influence deriving from his emotional self-control was the major factor. It was abetted in no small measure by the fact that he also kept the department's books. Keeping your head (and the books) when all others have lost theirs is the very essence of character strength in action.

3. Loss of Control of Affects

Arrogance. We must grant that the arrogant are sometimes smarter or stronger in some ways than many of the people around them. Their character flaw manifests itself in their belief that they are thereby worthier and more entitled to life's benefits. They fail to see that with greater gifts come greater responsibilities, among which is the common decency of curbing the need to demonstrate superiority. This is, of course, extremely difficult if you are afflicted with a mood disorder that pushes you into displays of grandiosity exacerbated by cycles of low self-esteem. Good medical treatment is often a necessary precondition of curbing these displays. But medicine alone will not provide the empathy, the gratitude, and the sense of responsibility that must be cultivated by those who are not content merely to be gifted but who are committed to spiritual growth. They have been given gifts whose fruits are all the sweeter for benefiting rather than depriving others.

Envy. The green-eyed monster is such a plague on our house that it immediately wipes out any vestige of a spiritual life. Having just curbed arrogance, we are now confronted with colleagues and classmates who have done so much better than we have. They hold eminent positions, have written books of renown, have made important scientific discoveries, or own beautiful villas in the south of France. Our first impulse is to trash them. The book wasn't so great, the discovery was really stolen from a lab assistant, and how ostentatious to own a villa in decadent old Europe!

But truly, if they were free of charge, who wouldn't want these accomplishments and riches? And why can't we give our colleagues their due? There are several issues. The first is the matter of talent. Do we have the requisite abilities to write a really good book or make a pioneering discovery? Is this our real purpose in life? Would we really change places with those who have achieved notoriety and be willing to expend the effort necessary to meet the attendant demands on our time and resources? Given our own temperament and talents, the distortions in the shape of our lives might be unbearable. Of course, we may have the talent but have not realized our potential, in which case we should cultivate the generosity of spirit to extend admiration to those who have realized theirs. But more importantly, we must examine very closely how they did it and see to what extent we can emulate them. Where feasible, we must move from envy to admiration and emulation.

The envy that does not lead to inspiration and resolve to do better ourselves virtually destroys all chance of having a spiritual life. Along with paranoia and heartless perfectionism, envy is a great soul-murderer. It poisons every opportunity to enjoy and admire the handiwork of our fellow human beings, who no longer share a common self but have become alien rivals.

For example, Mr. B had to give up hiking in his neighborhood because his neighbors' cars and houses made him so envious that he could not take in the fresh air and admire the beautiful designs of the gardens and the architecture all around him. He was an obsessive-compulsive perfectionist who refused to take medicine to soften these personality trends. He tried to solve his problem by looking only at his feet and counting his steps when he hiked, but he kept bumping into the trees and stones lining the path. His personal rigidity precluded an expansive experience of life's riches, shared in some way by us all. Fortunately, he was able to learn to enjoy foreign travel, where envy was less easily triggered.

4. Passivity and Regression

Sloth. This richly suggestive word for laziness and passivity captures the blob-like inertia of those who hold nothing worth fighting for except vegetative comfort. I once knew a man who owned a retail business in a small town. Besides an advanced case of gluttony—he weighed over four hundred pounds—he never moved from his stool behind the cash register. When customers asked for certain items, he directed them to the appropriate aisle, whose stock his wife and daughter maintained. He actually had the customers wrap their own items long before the days of self-service stores. Only the hand that operated the cash register ever got any exercise. On the weekends, his wife chauffeured him around while he sat in the backseat gorging on very large salamis and many bottles of cola. He rested up from his strenuous labors by taking restorative naps. His wife's account of how they made love, which she needed little encouragement to relate, was rich in its one-sided detail.

Bizarre as this story might seem, it is not so far removed from the common scenario of present-day men, women, and children spending whole nights and weekends glued to the television set. While watching sporting events, game shows, and sitcoms, we consume quantities of junk food to manage the anxious thrill of confronting the "dangerous" uncertainties of the high-risk situations we are viewing. Fortunately, such inactivity may keep some of us out of worse trouble, like stealing and cheating. But what we are not doing is strengthening our character, developing the disciplined activity that serves as a gymnastics of body and soul.

The Program

The program to build character strength is very simple to define. First, destructive internal saboteurs that undermine the will to health and creativity must be identified, corralled, and co-opted. We discussed how this is done in chapters 4 and 5, which address the subjects of the divided will and how it is integrated and activated. Second, we must overcome the passivity and excesses typified by the deadly sins. The patient must undertake a series of will-strengthening exercises aimed at curbing excesses and promoting active striving. This is the royal road to realizing one's potential. What must be determined first is whether or not there is an intact core will—that is, the capacity to act purposively. This is tested out by giving the patient homework to do.

Homework. Obviously, the most basic homework task is to show up for appointments at the scheduled time and place. By definition, the inability to do this precludes a voluntary outpatient therapy, even more a job, because there is demonstrably too little capacity for keeping schedules or promises. The next issue is compliance with the treatment regimen, whether this be taking medications at the prescribed time and dosage or following psychodynamic directives (e.g., reporting dreams, slips, and embarrassing feelings) or cognitive-behavioral directives (e.g., anxiety-exposure, positive thinking). It sometimes helps to have an external observer, such as a parent or partner, to validate these issues of compliance. Otherwise, in our permissive culture, therapist and patient are prone to develop the *folie a deux* that treatment is progressing when nothing significant beyond social intercourse is happening. Sometimes types of homework can be assigned that serve as holograms of the patient's total inability to progress. These are particularly helpful when patients appear to be cooperating but are making no progress in reaching their goals.

For example, Lloyd was a forty-eight-year-old research assistant doing important original work on animal behavior. Because he never published any of his data (which did not prevent his colleagues from drawing on his findings), he could not be promoted. What work he was able to do was all done in the spring and summer, when he became extremely active and energetic. Come fall, he became lethargic and slept many hours a day, often calling in sick. When he was put on lithium carbonate, his energy level and mood evened out, but he still couldn't focus on writing up his findings. He said he felt blocked. When he laid out his data sheets, his mind went blank. We explored relevant biological and psychosocial factors and the remedies suggested by our findings, but still no progress was made.

Drawing on a will-testing technique of the Italian psychiatrist Roberto Assagioli,[79] I suggested to Lloyd that he could overcome his block if he would only stand on a chair every morning for five minutes and report to me what he experienced. Despite avidly agreeing to follow this directive, he complied only once. Either he forgot or was too late for work, or he encountered some other obstacle. I knew then that a therapy based on a cooperative will was, for the time being, out of the question. Whether the culprit was an internal saboteur, repressed rage, psychotic oppositionalism, or some subtle brain defect, his inability to carry out this seemingly trivial exercise ruled out further progress by the means at our disposal. He seemingly had no core will to develop, no voluntary muscle to pump iron with, at least in the time we had together.

<u>Anchoring the Will</u>. Once the patient demonstrates the capacity to act willfully, the will must be anchored. By this I mean that it must be fastened firmly to daily routines that provide traction for exerting other, more difficult feats of self-control. For example, alcoholics are sometimes enabled to abstain from drinking if they attend an AA meeting faithfully every day or several times daily. The process is further buttressed by reporting to a sponsor at regular times. Once sobriety is established, then the mental and physical rituals involved in resisting the urge to drink are used as anchors to desist from other self-destructive acts. For example, a three-times-divorced thirty-four-year-old ex-alcoholic who was about to run out on her best-ever relationship

was enjoined to use the same discipline involved in maintaining sobriety to resist the urge to provoke another breakup. She was responsive to the notion that curbing the impulse to drink was far easier than curbing her fear of attachment and consequent flight.

The heaviest anchor is a daily exercise routine. This must be initiated in the proper spirit: one must stake one's life on adhering to the routine, no matter if one has eaten or drunk too much or slept too little, or bad weather prohibits going outside. The big mistake most people make in choosing an exercise anchor is choosing one that takes too much time or is too hard to do. Trendsetters in these matters are often perfectionists whose determination either borders on the pathological or exceeds the capacities of ordinary people. What is needed is a manageable program, as short as fifteen to thirty minutes a day, that can be done regularly, rain or shine. Vigorous walking, outdoors or in a mall or on a treadmill, is the most universally applicable exercise; but jogging, doing stomach crunches and push-ups, swimming laps, or using various exercise machines may be the right thing depending on the individual's particular needs and capacities. What is important is that the time required and the degree of difficulty not constitute intimidating factors in getting it done. Within reasonable limits, the regularity, rather than the time and difficulty, is what really counts. Of course, more vigorous programs are appropriate for the athletically inclined who can make the time.

Once the basic routine is established, then it can be used as leverage to extend self-control to other areas of life. As everyone knows but tries to forget, gluttony and obesity are best overcome by, in addition to an exercise program, proper food selection and portion control. The dietary rituals required to succeed here are a very individual matter, dependent on personal needs and tastes. But rituals there must be, and they must be enacted with the same religious devotion as the exercise program, which serves as the primary anchor. Keeping kosher; becoming a vegetarian; avoiding bread, desserts, and pastas; limiting red meats and simple carbohydrates; taking home half of main portions from restaurants—these are some of the many routines that successful dieters have used to get their eating and weight under control.

Similarly, for each of the excesses embodied in the other deadly sins, rituals must be found and adhered to as the means of strengthening character and will. The rageful must learn anger-management techniques, which involve identifying trigger situations and developing alternative, constructive forms of aggression. Successful routines abound for curbing sexual desire and other problematic needs as well. The "how to" is less the problem than the "must do." Individuals with character flaws rarely see the necessity of taking action to repair their defects. They do not foresee the terrible destiny that their weak character is generating. Once they are made fully aware of it, half the battle is over, and finding the right techniques comes more easily. Breaking through the barrier of resistance, to blow the cover of saboteurs and rein in out-of-control drives and needs, is greatly furthered by becoming a member of a spiritual group capable of giving corrective feedback in a tough-love mode. But there is no substitute for intuitive therapists with artistic skills in implementing effective programs. Finding effective, personally tailored routines and getting people to stake their lives on following them is crucial to the art of psychotherapy. Success here is intimately bound up with the therapist's capacity for empathy, which along with character constitutes the essence of the spirituality of patient and therapist. The influence of these capacities is immeasurably aided by the ability to paint a dramatic picture of the consequences of an undisciplined life deficient in guiding spiritual ideals.

Chapter 9
EMPATHY

Summary. I discuss the role of compassionate empathy in the development of spirituality and particularly the differential contributions of character and empathy to spiritualizing the lives of individuals and communities. I emphasize the strenuous effort required to develop these qualities, no matter how strong their natural endowment. We fix the good into our character by repeatedly choosing to act morally, as Maimonides maintained, but such choices are rarely made without personal sacrifice. The faculties of intuition and critical thinking fortify our compassionate empathy and, even more broadly, direct us to perceive and apply the principles of the moral law in all aspects of our daily lives. In the process we have the opportunity to develop the rudimentary soul we are born with into a higher self that can unite with the all-embracing Soul that I call Spirit. The process of allowing Spirit to pervade our lives is arduous but crucial to leading a spiritual life, to living right. We are blessed to live at a time when, with the help of medical science and spiritual care, we can realize Maimonides's noble ideal—by first repairing our free will and then using it, step by step, to develop character and empathy, in the process experiencing the opportunity to identify with Spirit.

Developing a spiritual life, as distinguished from following the practices of formal religion, crucially depends on developing both character and empathy. Character provides the basic infrastructure of spirituality. Without its firm foundation, spiritual passion can easily explode into the dark storms of cultism and fanaticism. Character is essential to keeping spirituality grounded in the causality of everyday spatiotemporal life.

In its absence we encounter the likes of the already mentioned Indian guru Bhagwan Shree Rajneesh, writer of many books on spiritual topics.[80] Unfortunately, he began to feel worthy of the adulation of his followers and fostered their attempt to take over the county government adjacent to his compound in rural Oregon. His grandiose labeling of his messianic lawlessness as a "cosmic joke" did not deter local and federal authorities from expelling Baghwan from the country. Claims of cosmic insight crumble in the absence of a solid foundation of good character.

Yet however much it is needed to ground spirituality, character alone will not give access to the higher reaches of Spirit. Character operates to a significant degree in the realm of ordinary empirical consciousness, where you and I are bound by mutual obligations, and we are all bound together by the social contract, which guarantees our freedoms and the rule of law. This arrangement is predicated on our being held accountable as separate people with individual traits and beliefs trying to live together in harmony despite having conflicting needs. In this everyday world, we count on our friends and colleagues to keep their word, to stand by us in hard times, and to show reciprocal appreciation of our gifts and requirements. And in return for our taxes and good citizenship, the society owes us a range of judicial and civil services and, above all, security from unlawful aggression. To the extent that we are of sound character, we are always mindful of these personal and social obligations. Character enters the spiritual realm when we stand firm in our loyalties to people and institutions and obedience to the universal moral principles, sometimes at the cost of great personal suffering even unto death.

The exercise of empathy, in contrast to character, moves more decisively beyond ordinary consciousness into the realm of intuitive spiritual awareness. With empathy we are able to perceive what others are thinking and feeling, often with the help of their body language, but sometimes aided only by an imaginative evocation of their character and interests. In the most developed states of empathic attunement, we directly experience the experience of others, seemingly beyond the contribution of sensory experience. In competitive situations, such empathic knowing can give ruthless parties a significant advantage in bending others to their will. Yet this partial empathy does not prove decisive in helping them identify with others to the extent of caring about them.

Caring empathy is empathy combined with sympathy. Sympathetic or compassionate empathy, the kind that concerns us here, occurs when feeling what others are feeling is accompanied by feeling *for* them. It is a way of knowing that transcends our senses and our separateness. In this highest state of empathic attunement, the distinction between you and me is at least partially obliterated, so that, to some degree, "I am you" and "you are we." The *Bhagavad-Gita*,[81] a seminal work in Hindu mysticism, goes so far as to say that in the highest state of unitive consciousness, "That art thou!" Here the separation between the self and the entire material world is seen to be illusory. Self and object and I and thou are all *One*. Everyone and everything are mere projections or outpocketings of a single all-embracing consciousness.

To appreciate and demonstrate caring empathy in the spiritual life does not require us to go so far. But we must go far enough to recognize that such attunement allows us to experience the feelings, thoughts, and wishes of others and, even if only at special times, to care about what happens to them as much as what happens to us. For most, this identification occurs only in the most exalted states, as when we are deeply in love. In loving empathy, we directly share in our loved ones' attitudes and feelings, so that we can truly say that we take joy in their joy and pain from their pain. Beyond romantic partners, we see this most clearly in the unconditional love sometimes found between parents and children and most strikingly between intimately related identical twins. In some twins, the mutual resonance of mental states can be so complete that the individuals involved have unequivocally generated a common self.

To conventional psychopathologists, such alleged phenomena of unitive consciousness are diagnosable as illusions or even psychotic delusions. From this vantage point, individual minds are closed systems with no access to one another except through the data of ordinary sense perception. To think otherwise, as schizophrenics do when they claim direct access to the will and thoughts of others, as in "thought-broadcasting" and delusions of control and influence, is no less pathological than believing in extraterrestrial beings or hovering spirits of the dead. Parapsychologists have a different take on these phenomena. They believe that some claims of nonsensory psychic influence are legitimate, deriving from so-called extrasensory perception and psychokinesis, about which they claim to have scientific evidence.[82]

Whatever the merits of the work of parapsychologists—I obviously believe in some of their conclusions but do not as yet accept the validity of their scientific "proofs"—the spiritual therapist believes in a more comprehensive formulation: namely, that individual minds can aggregate into larger wholes: group minds or spirits. When this happens, each one of us can function as a holographic cell or microcosm of a larger tissue of mind, so that the individual gains access to and reflects the whole, with its creative and healing powers and also, as LeBon and Freud recognized, its potentially destructive powers. The spiritualization of a therapeutic group that gains these positive potentials and curbs the negative ones, already touched upon, will be further elaborated in the next chapter.

When we participate in a larger group self, we can bridge the gap between "us" and "them" by intuitions, related to what Daniel Kahneman calls fast thinking and Malcolm Gladwell calls blinks: heightened perceptions about other people and circumstances that turn out to be accurate representations of intentions and what is about to happen or has already happened.[83] For example, an identical twin, having the thought that it is time to make contact, dials her twin sister only to discover that she is already on the line, obviating an audible ring. This is a frequent occurrence with the twins. Or someone has an out-of-the-blue sense of foreboding, only subsequently to discover that a loved one simultaneously had a near-fatal accident. Almost as uncannily, a point guard with "high basketball IQ" anticipates the direction, speed, and movement patterns of each member of his basketball team, so that he can make the perfect alley-oop or backdoor pass for a score. Is this just familiarity with individual tendencies, signals, and highly rehearsed plays, or does it go beyond ordinary perception to tap into an intuited *esprit de corps*, a single group mind, as when a flock of birds takes flight instantaneously in perfect formation? I believe the latter possibility is often at work, even though we must always be ready to use Occam's razor if simpler, naturalistic explanations can be shown to account for the phenomena.[84]

The Psychotic versus the Spiritual

The biggest conundrum facing this supra-sensory line of thought is the difficulty in distinguishing spiritual phenomena from psychotic symptoms. Perhaps we can clarify the situation by distinguishing psychosis and spirituality from the syndromes with which they overlap and are often confused: primary process thinking and infantile symbiosis. By psychosis we mean the state of being out of touch with everyday reality. Delusions and hallucinations are primary indicators of this loss of contact with reality, as are the bizarre, symbolic behaviors inspired by them. For example, a patient repeatedly and dramatically falls to the floor as he marches about the ward. He claims to be Jesus Christ descending from the cross. "Bizarre," "grandiose," "messianic," and "histrionic" are some of the adjectives we invoke to indicate our belief that the individual is no longer anchored in everyday reality.

By convention, incoherent, noncausal thinking and inappropriate or flat affect are also common manifestations of psychosis. We say that such individuals have severe thought and mood disorders. As a result they are prone to social breakdown: the state of being disorganized to the point that self-care and ability to work productively are compromised. They also manifest porous and fluid sensory and structural boundaries: their minds are easily penetrated by the attitudes and feelings of others, and they often betray an insufficiently developed sense of privacy and ownership, manifested by inappropriately sharing their inner thoughts and giving away their possessions. When conversing, they stand too close to us or touch us too familiarly and think they are helping us by giving us a "free" analysis of our motives. In short, they frequently, without invitation, invade the mental and physical space of others. Their porous boundaries make them vulnerable to losing their separate identities and taking on the attributes of individuals and groups, particularly those in authority or objects of fear or affection.

Note that the latter phenomenon of lost identity may be a constituent of but does not add up to psychosis all by itself. Lost identity may be part of broader cultural phenomena: for example, the irrational attitudes and beliefs shared by large segments of a population that totalitarian societies typically enforce, exemplified by the widespread "willing executioners" of the Final Solution of Hitler's Germany and the anti-intellectual Cultural Revolution of Mao's China.

Primary process thinking is characterized by regressive thinking, experience, and behavior that are not bound by considerations of logic, causality, and propriety. As a result, primary process is drenched in images of highly charged primitive activities, such as having a sexual orgy in a cave covered with bloody animal skins, as one of my patients imagined. As an example of another type of primary process, Doris, a highly trained medical professional, thought that by marrying Sam, a thirty-two-year-old uneducated recovering alcoholic working in a low-paying job, she would gain a suitable husband and father to her child if she only paid for his college education and therapy. She could not see beyond their mutual infatuation to recognize that his uncontrolled addictive and impulsive behavior—as previously mentioned, he actually broke into her bank account to buy books and expensive food and cigars—would have made him a candidate for jail time had he not been restrained by genuine remorse over his theft and other violations of the moral code. The element of magical thinking involved in Doris's decision making takes it beyond mere bad judgment to the irrationality of primary process thinking.

In infantile symbiosis, children do not individuate from their mothers to develop a fully formed separate identity. To the extent that they have a self at all, it is a fused self identified for the most part with the needs and capacities of their caretakers. The great Hungarian mathematician Paul Erdos was carried in his mother's arms well into his late teens. When asked by a colleague at a professional meeting why Paul didn't walk on his own, his mother replied, "Because he doesn't have to." After she died, Erdos lived out of suitcases, making the rounds of collaborators' homes, often arriving without prior warning, where the women of the house fed him and did his laundry. The vast majority of his papers were jointly authored, perhaps further evidence of his lack of an individuated self.

The lack of a fully formed independent self, with the attendant personal boundary disturbance suggestive of underlying psychosis, is the symbiotic's most salient feature. A less severe, adult form is dependent personality, in which the individual is submissive to the thoughts and wishes of dominant people in their lives. The individual can barely function socially in their absence. At its extreme, such people manifest the neurotic and even psychotic attitudes of their leaders. They have "escaped from freedom," in Erich Fromm's memorable phrase,[85] to succumb to *folie a deux*, group-think, or becoming moral captives of totalitarian regimes.

Spirituality Again

By personal spirituality, we mean that the self manifests the phenomena indicative of having a soul—that is, of participating in the workings of a common higher consciousness: Spirit. By recognizing the binding truth of the moral code, which enjoins us not only to treat others as we would have them treat us but also to behave righteously toward ourselves and the world, we become spiritual to the extent that our recognition goes beyond expediency to an empathetic appreciation of our common being, our shared universe of consciousness. Similarly, appreciating the near-universality of certain standards of moral and aesthetic beauty is of the very essence of spirituality, allowing people growing up in China to be moved by a Beethoven symphony or a Shakespearean sonnet. On a more personal moral level, having a soul means that we are moved by every hungry or abused child, by every tortured or oppressed fellow human being, by every one of Hurricane Katrina's drowned or homeless victims. We compassionately empathize with them so that we suffer on their behalf and try to extend our charity to agencies of social and spiritual repair.

The Vulnerability of Spirituality

The porousness and fluidity of boundaries required to achieve empathic identification makes the spiritual person vulnerable to both primary process thinking and psychosis, where the wish can become grandiosely delusional and trump the sense of the appropriate. Think of the young heir of a grocery chain fortune handing out $100 bills on a street corner some years back. Was this evidence of something more than unanchored guilt and grandiosity? I believe so, but the underlying spiritual impulse was obscured by the individual's bizarre manifestations of his tenuous hold on everyday reality. Spirituality can also shade into symbiotic psychosis, where individual identity is drowned in a sea of human distress or proselytizing messianism. Yet healthy individuals can be spiritual without succumbing to symbiosis, psychosis, or primary process. They accomplish this through their flexibility to maintain parallelism between the states of empathetic identification and self-protective individuality.

Dipping into empathetic, spiritual awareness allows us to see the whole, to appreciate our common humanity and purpose. Staying there, without the tempering effect of everyday subject-object awareness, will just as surely drive us mad because, in sustained heightened awareness, we cannot integrate all that we undeniably see and feel. To avert this outcome, characteristic of psychedelic-induced spiritual states and misapplications of "Eastern wisdom" to naïve "Western truth seeking," the individual must be able to maintain a dual consciousness—to use an accounting metaphor, the individual must keep two sets of books—and alternate between the common-spiritual and individual-sensible modes as prompted by circumstances. As I shall discuss later, a form of dissociation is a vital component of this capacity.

Sane Spirituality

In sum, we distinguish integrated spiritual persons, those with a functioning creative soul, from psychotics by the fact that they are socially functional and have the capacity to reconstitute their individual self at will. This they are able to do after immersions in heightened, unitive awareness. Those who cannot, having found it too difficult to reconstitute boundaries after spiritual experience, are doomed to suffering psychotic ego disintegration in its aftermath. In states of physical and spiritual union, we momentarily throw off the coils of individuality. This is the so-called death of the ego.

Afterwards, our boundaries and identities are restored as we reenter the everyday spatiotemporal world.

Individuals who have intimations of spiritual awareness but who cannot make the transitions between the spiritual and the sensible smoothly, who cannot maintain alternating, dual consciousness, manifest various psychiatric disorders, typically borderline and psychotic states. For example, borderline personalities are notorious for instability of personal relationships. They may abruptly break off seemingly close friendships because of sudden changes of feelings. Sometimes love turns on a dime into hate, or comfort with the other turns into fear of engulfment or annihilation. They feel forced to bolt rather than ride out the ego-threatening storms intrinsic to passionate closeness. They cannot stand firm in their affections and loyalties. In an understatement of the obvious, we say that they have problems with intimacy. Similarly, those who manifest inhibited libido, we typically characterize as sexually repressed and plagued by guilt. But in many cases these formulations do not go far enough. Beyond repression and guilt, spiritual borderlines may suffer from fragility and rigidity of character. They cannot oscillate between the empathic consciousness of spiritual union and the ordinary consciousness of individual identity without either shutting down and withdrawing or falling apart. For example, a gifted poet with borderline psychotic symptoms said she dare not make love with her paramour because the last time she achieved orgasm with him, she felt her sense of self "splatter all over the ceiling." She felt disintegrated and unable to function for days afterward and only gradually glued herself back together by compulsively cleaning house and rearranging clothes and furniture.

We conclude that some individuals cannot sustain intimate connections and cannot fully achieve sexual and spiritual union because these potentially unitive states threaten the integrity of the empirical self. They cannot reconstitute their ego boundaries after union and therefore may have to resort to distancing techniques rather than risk uncontrolled immersion in the ego dissolution of the spiritual, unitive state. Treatments that provide flexible "psychic glue," such as psychoactive medication and carefully executed organizing rituals—cleaning the house, straightening the desk, making regular social plans, and keeping to a schedule are common examples—may contribute to making it possible for such people to stay more closely attached while maintaining the ability to function in the everyday world. More fundamentally, they must be helped to appreciate their spiritual gifts and the dangers the gifts expose them to without adequate preparation, part of which is a facility in controlled, creative dissociation.

Creative Dissociation

As we have often discussed, defensive dissociation is the patient's way of avoiding psychosis when assaulted by unbearable physical and psychological trauma. This maneuver has the unintended consequences of sequestering psychic energy and creating internal saboteurs. By means of defensive dissociation, we split in order not to shatter, but as indicated the costs are high. The process usually occurs automatically and outside conscious control, much as a circuit breaker shuts down the electrical supply to avoid frying the circuitry of appliances.

Our mental appliances can also be saved by conscious dissociation to mitigate the ego-destroying effects of an unprepared immersion in spiritual awareness. In the "Allegory of the Cave," Plato called the mitigating process habituation. Compartmentalization is another popular term used to describe a part of the process. Under conscious control by gradual exposure, it can be used to gain access to Spirit on enhancing rather than destructive terms. Rather than unconsciously splitting off some of our spiritual energy and risk diverting its power into a saboteur, we only temporarily sideline it while we take care of everyday business. Rather than risking a potentially mind-blowing immersion in Spirit, this kind of dissociation can be therapeutic rather than pathological, particularly if we can summon it at will rather than have it forced on us. Therapeutic splitting allows us to have a spiritual life without losing our moorings in empirical reality and without forming a self-defeating part of the self such as an internal saboteur. And in fact, therapeutic dissociation is what I was alluding to in speaking of an oscillation between empathic unitive and individual empirical consciousness: flexibly splitting our attention between two different states of awareness, two different accounts and ways of experiencing reality.

Conventionally religious people accomplish this therapeutic dissociation by confining their spiritual life for the most part to daily mass or Sabbath attendance at church or synagogue and setting regular times for private prayer. In a prescribed way, they focus their attention at these times on entreaties and gratitude for divine intercession and meditations on the classic spiritual questions: what is my relationship to a higher power, why am I suffering and what should I do to prevent or overcome it, and how can I find contentment? The goal of a spiritual therapy, in contrast, is to be connected continuously to the higher reality, Spirit, which transforms these questions into intuited wisdom that transcends the need for concrete answers. Rather than importuning a deity outside ourselves, we locate the Spirit within us, and uniting with it becomes the reason and purpose of everything: our existence and the existence of the world and everything in it, with its cycles of life and death and epiphanous joys and devastating sorrows. Rather than once a day or once a week, the oscillation or parallelism between the spiritual and the sensible is ongoing. Instead of concretizing the sense of the ineffable and the holy into a conception of a God who intervenes in our daily lives, the spiritual person is likely to strive to feel united with an all-embracing, organizing, and caring Will, focused not on our individual needs but on realizing our universal ideals. Yet in trying to align ourselves with the flow of willful Spirit, we must remain mindful of our everyday obligations, remembering to pick up the children after school and to pay the bills.

Focusing Attention

How to achieve this parallel consciousness is one of the most important teachings of the spiritual therapist. It involves the ability to focus attention so sharply that it becomes itself an all-conquering creative will—in fact, a powerful multitasking will capable of cutting through all obstacles erected by the egocentric, objective self. A hologram of this task can be found in the breathing meditation. If we focus our attention exclusively on a point behind the sternum as we engage in diaphragmatic breathing, we soon become increasingly aware of the various phenomena involved in the intake and expulsion of breath; we see that among these are two fundamental components: involuntary biorhythmic breathing and voluntary interventional breathing. The latter can be summoned to override the former to meet exceptional situations, such as having to swim fast underwater or deal with dangerous smoke or gas leaks. In ordinary situations the task is to coordinate the two types of breathing so that they work together instead of against each other; the latter often happens in states of hyper-willfulness. In these states of high anxiety and obsessive-compulsion, we tend to override the body's automatic regulatory mechanisms; we overbreathe in a shallow gasping manner that creates a vicious cycle of apnea and hyperventilation—all in desperate hunger for the sustaining spiritual breath, the soul's life force.

Once we achieve the depth of focus that facilitates harmonious deep breathing, where the involuntary and the voluntary are synchronized and all distractions are banished, then we have achieved the altered state of consciousness conducive to experiencing the simultaneity of Spirit and sense, of internal will and external cause, of immaterial, spiritual reality and material, objective reality. This split awareness not only gives us knowledge of two realms of truth, but also gives us the power to modify-align our empirical reality with the spiritual reality and, conversely, to temper our spiritual experiences so that they do not incapacitate us from managing the demands of everyday living. Without this capacity for therapeutic dissociation, we can be blown away into mini-psychosis by direct spiritual experience, for the capacity to recover our everyday functioning depends on our ability to switch back from the spiritual into the material mode of perception as needed.

For some of us, to avoid the risk to sanity posed by awe-inspiring, numinous experiences, we may have to renounce their sacred meaning at least for the period of time required to integrate them with our empirical mindset. For example, after great successes or narrow brushes with death, we might be tempted to assign the cause of our deliverance to a supernatural agency that has focused its beneficence exclusively on our welfare. The narcissism and grandiosity of such thinking exposes the dangers of becoming too attached and residing too long in the intuitive, spiritual mode without touching base with everyday empirical awareness. Rather than leaping to such far-fetched conclusions, we would be better served to confine our reactions to states of bemused wonderment.

When spiritual awareness cannot be integrated into the everyday worldview, the renunciation of its truths is more typically accomplished by repression and denial, or by diagnosing these experiences as pathological. At their most obnoxiously reductive, epiphany deniers can issue hostile condemnations of anyone, patient and stranger alike, who affirms a belief in the existence of any powers higher than human intellect and blind chance.

Preparations for Spiritual Immersion

In recognition of the dangers of spiritual immersion for the unprepared mind, every great religious tradition has preparatory disciplines for delving into it. In the Judaic tradition, noteworthy for being grounded in the everyday world, seekers after higher truth are specifically forbidden to approach the mystical-spiritual core of faith until they reach the age of emotional maturity, get married, and study the Torah everyday. Without these grounding structures, the great rabbis recognized the occupational hazard of losing one's connections to sanity and society in the spiritual quest.

In the ecumenical spiritual therapy approach, a healthy mode of unitive, empathic experience can be achieved under less restrictive conditions provided that essential prerequisites are met and the search is undertaken in good faith. But we must not imagine that the work is ever less than arduous. To start with, depressive psychosis and paranoid psychosis, two of the greatest distorters of spiritual perception, must be rigorously combatted, especially since they are also the most serious casualties of the spiritual quest. In the absence of marriage and Torah study, equivalent grounding structures must be developed, such as a strong relationship network and a disciplined course of study and work in a mainstream field of knowledge. To satisfy this latter condition, we should be wary of using alternative medicine approaches, even well-established ones such as yoga and acupuncture, as the sole partnering disciplines since their grounding in Western culture, of such recent vintage, is subject to the distortions of trendy enthusiasm.

The Work of Therapeutic Dissociation

Once the individual's psychobiological equipment has been put in working order through alleviation of depression and paranoia and other mood and thought disorders, the ability to alternate and parallel successfully between the sensible and the spiritual perspectives requires specialized development in three major areas of experience. First, we must unearth the conditions of early life hostile to the child's burgeoning spirituality. Second, we must undertake the empathetic and cognitive retraining required to overcome this developmental block. And third, once it is reclaimed and developed, we must learn to interiorize and channel our intuitive-empathic access to spiritual truth.

1. The Traumatic Loss of Empathy in Early Life

Most children come into the world with natural capacities for empathy and spiritual connection, which are all too easily blighted by an inhospitable environment. As the boy becomes the man (and the girl the woman), the gift of spiritual love often becomes degraded. Loss of parents, withdrawal of love, physical and sexual abuse, repeated humiliations—these all cause deep scarring on the thin skin of heightened sensibility.

In recent years, self psychology has reclaimed the nineteenth-century emphasis on dissociation, as opposed to Freudian repression, as a prime etiology of neurotic behavior. In my account of the internal saboteur, I have borrowed heavily from this approach. According to it, when a sensitive child is traumatized by physical or sexual abuse, the overwhelming emotional pain that results is blunted by the pain-bearing part of the self splitting off from central awareness. This dissociation functions as a circuit breaker, thereby sparing the self a psychotic burnout. In the process, an uncontrolled partial self is formed, which not only carries the hurt and anger caused by the initial trauma but which also soaks ups ambient hostility from the environment. By identification, the enraged, destructive partial self becomes a magnet for the negative qualities of all abusers, torturers, and persecutors the person encounters, particularly in the family environment, but also from esteemed political and religious leaders. In the process, the resultant internal saboteur comes to carry not only the hurt and rage of being abused but also the rage of the abusers, reinforced by ambient experiences and accompanying ideologies. It identifies with the aggressor in a very broad sense.

For example, Penny is a social worker who first consulted me in the aftermath of a postpartum depression followed by sexual promiscuity and divorce. Raised by harsh Southern bigots (her mother had been a gruff sergeant in the Women's Army Corps in World War II), Penny had tried to escape the daily drill by defecating and urinating in the backyard. When after college she declared her intention of becoming a social worker, her parents railed that she would only be "helping the N's live off the government." After a family conference, she asked her parents for financial help in paying for her treatment. The money came but not without the admonition that she was "just helping that Jew doctor get rich."

Drawing on a basic sense of decency, Penny fought to become a generous helping person with integrity of character. Her intake evaluations, which she asked me to critique, were some of the most sensitive and compassionate that

I have encountered in a long experience of supervising health professionals. In her own group therapy, she displayed an unerring instinct for spotting and supporting admirable traits in others. She befriended a fellow member, a liberal rabbi, whom she asked to officiate at her nonsectarian remarriage. The look on her mother's face at the wedding would surely qualify as one of the most puke-faced moments in modern psychotherapy.

Yet the ravages of Penny's upbringing left deep holes in her soul. She could not ordinarily enjoy the physical act of love—never with her devoted husband, only when she had been drunk and promiscuous with strangers or men of dubious character. A mean voice inside her said that sex was lowdown and dirty, meant only for N's and J's. Similarly, when she did her artwork (she was an accomplished fabric artist), the inner voice said that she was wasting her time; she should be out doing practical work. Sometimes, when fellow group members complained or showed vulnerabilities similar to her own, she would become harshly judgmental, adopting the taunting voice of her mother while hurling epithets of bigoted condemnation. The counterattack to these outbursts, even the attempt to explain the workings of her saboteur in their production, initially brought loud sobs and attempts to run out of the office, as Penny instantly shifted from playing the harsh mother to being the wounded, misunderstood child. Even more bizarrely, she could not allow herself to listen to music or go to museums despite having a natural appreciation for all the visual and performance arts. She was comfortable only viewing and working with quilts and other art pieces that had a utilitarian purpose. Her overt spiritual life was confined to ruminations about the meaninglessness of life and her own sinfulness.

In such a case, we see the workings of a traumatic upbringing in producing a split-off tormentor that attacked her and others instead of allowing for a measure of pleasure and empathy. The voice of the tormenting saboteur was an alloy of the voices of her Southern, bigoted parents and the fundamentalist preachers who had guided her early religious education. Her natural spirituality, evidenced by her religious and racial tolerance, charitable giving, identification with the underdog, and exquisite moral and aesthetic sensitivity, was blighted to the point that she could not freely enjoy artistic expression or generate a creative and healing belief system: one that gave meaning to her life, that allowed her to use her profession to help others.

2. The Trauma of Empathic Deficiency in Parents

The blunting of spirituality, indeed of intuitive-empathic feelings in general, is quite understandable in cases of physical and emotional abuse. But we often find the anti-spiritual and destructive workings of split-off saboteurs in the absence of any history of ostensible abuse. Try as we might to find evidence, even bringing into the office impartial witnesses of patients' past lives, we fail to elicit corroborative evidence of obvious trauma, leaving us mystified as to the cause of dissociation. What is the possible explanation for the mystery?

What we often find in these cases is an alignment of two special circumstances: a child who is uncommonly sensitive and gifted and parents whose self fabric is too insensitive for them to appreciate their child's special qualities. The children in such cases experience not the usual kinds of trauma but the devastation of the emotional rebuff that follows the exuberant manifestation of their gifts—a variation on the theme of "casting pearls before swine." Well fed, clothed, and sheltered, they are nevertheless left feeling unsupported and wounded; they feel exposed and pierced for saying and doing what limited parents think of as ridiculous arrogance, for behavior that evokes detached neglect or even ridicule. Humiliation, mortification, narcissistic injury, punctured grandiosity—these are some of the terms used to characterize the traumatic effect of nonempathetic parents on spiritually gifted children.

For example, Doris, most of whose close relationships involved highly inappropriate men, culminating in the already mentioned disastrous marriage to Sam, gave no history of overt trauma in forming her split-off love saboteur. In fact, at a family conference, her parents seemed to be good people who wanted to do the right thing. But they were emotionally detached. Her mother, in particular, despite saying all the right things, conveyed a puzzling objectivity, which I did not fully understand at the time. Doris, on the other hand, was brimming with warmth and affection and a unique capacity for spiritual and aesthetic expression—she was an uncommonly gifted singer and pianist, talents demonstrated at an early age—which her mother responded to correctly but without much enthusiasm, leading Doris to try ever more extreme measures to secure emotional approval. In contrast, Doris's sister, a more robustly extraverted type, was perpetually enraged, constantly screaming at her mother and accusing her of disinterest and favoritism toward Doris. In fact both girls were neglected emotionally. In spite of high achievement and personal attractiveness, Doris was left with a profound sense of inferiority and with a love saboteur that picked men who were either unavailable or intellectually and spiritually beneath her, and for whom she had barely hidden contempt. Unfortunately, some of them also exploited her.

For Doris to locate the origins of this acting-out part of the self, she had to see behind the always correct behavior of her parents and locate the traumatic pain caused by their empathic failure, particularly in one so profoundly loving and spiritual as herself. The split-off awareness of its impact was finally recaptured when one of her fellow group members, Sandy, accompanied Doris on a family visit. Upon her return to the group, Sandy expressed shock at how emotionally cold and detached her parents seemed, even when they played with Doris's baby, their grandson—a fact I had not fully appreciated at the family conference. This also helped me make sense of her difficulty in switching from the empathic to the objective mode in evaluating people: in the presence of attraction, becoming objectively evaluative was apparently too much like her parents' coolness, the possibility of which re-evoked the traumatic feelings associated with the splitting injury to her self-system. Sandy also observed on a social outing that Doris became coolly unresponsive when appropriate men approached her, which they often did—a striking exception to her warm response to most people. Obviously, there were inhibitions to loving an appropriate man, deriving in part from a disturbance in her relationship to her father as well as her mother. Doris interpreted her mother's coldness as a prohibition against showing affection toward her physician father and, by extension, toward any accomplished man.

In Doris's case, we see how a spiritually caring person is traumatized by emotionally unresponsive, nonempathic parents and how this leads to a love-thwarting internal saboteur. The experience also crippled Doris's ability to judge people accurately. Once she experienced sympathy for someone, whether in her personal or her professional life, she could not easily oscillate into the pragmatic, sensible mode and evaluate their motives and character—an inability that often came with disastrous results.

We can recognize children like Doris because they are obviously gifted. They show precocious language and artistic skills, often speaking in complete sentences, reading books, writing poems, or playing music long before the expected milestones of development. And often they have arresting perceptions and insights that lay matters bare, like asking if any other being has the same relationship to us as we have to household pets. As one gifted child asked, whose dogs and cats are we? They can be charmingly grandiose, laying claim to being great writers or painters with their very first productions. If they are shamed for these pretensions—in effect, told that they are too big for their britches—they feel deflated and can go on to experience the humiliation of punctured grandiosity, which if repeated often enough can result in permanent injury to the self, as evidenced by bouts of low self-esteem and the acting-out of a split-off saboteur.

These children not uncommonly speak of benevolent or hostile spirits—guardian angels and monsters in the night—that affect their lives. Sometimes they allude, all on their own, to a loving or angry God who is rewarding or punishing them. In doctrinaire atheistic families, such imaginings can be censured as absurd. Far from providing reassurance, these corrections, often spiced with ridicule, serve to discourage children from using their imaginative gifts to make sense of their experience. Even if their explanations are illusions, it is important to remember that the opposite of having them is to be disillusioned, as Otto Rank pointed out. Santa Claus should not be dispensed with prematurely.

Heinz Kohut, a Chicago psychoanalyst of the last century, believed that grandiosity is a separate developmental force, similar to but different from the sexual and aggressive instincts, that needs the taming effects of true appreciation and emotional support for the child to become an adult who shows empathic warmth and playful creativity.[86] Although I am indebted to this formulation, I believe it places the cart before the horse. The basic developmental force is a spiritual sensibility that is apparently grandiose because it tunes into the loving and creative force of all-consciousness like a finely tuned multichannel receiver. It is this holographic force, throbbing in the gifted child's soul, that gives the beat for its march toward mature forms of love and will. In the absence of sensitive listening and shaping, this spiritual beat can be thrown off, marching the gifted children, like lemmings, right off the cliff to spiritual death.

Empathetic and Cognitive Retraining

Once patients such as Doris gain access to the experiences responsible for the traumatic derailing of their spiritual gifts, they must be helped to recapture and develop them and especially to integrate them into the pragmatics of everyday living. In Doris's case this started with getting her to recognize that her warm empathy did not release her from the necessity of assessing the character and motivation of herself and others. In other words, she had to be urged repeatedly to be suspicious of her sympathy for others until she had undertaken an analysis of their intentions and reliability. In her work as a health professional and in her personal life, this meant that her caring response to the sufferings of patients and potential friends always had to be tempered by an appreciation of the realities of their situation, their character problems, their ability to cooperate, and the strength of their basic will to health and relationship. Otherwise she would always be in danger of investing too much of herself in lost causes or those that required special treatment and of being taken advantage of by those who typically take but do not give. After the assessment, she had to train herself to resist the blandishments of people who would most likely break her heart and to overcome her cool avoidance of the potentially worthy. Once she judged them to be appropriate candidates for a relationship, then she had to use all her gifts to make a claim on them. Over and over again, she had to be asked, "Who are you dealing with here [the diagnosis, the character assessment], what does the individual want, why do you like him, or why are you put off by her?"—until she could more easily perform these shifts of perspective on her own as she judged the feasibility of realizing her clinical or personal goals.

Helping Ordinary Individuals Reclaim Spirituality

What can be done for those with a low natural endowment of spiritual sensitivity? After the effects of mood and thought disorders and inhibiting past experiences are ameliorated, the retraining process involves a constant focus on instances of deficient character and empathy. Here effective therapy becomes more obviously a form of moral treatment, of training in applied ethics. Patients are repeatedly asked if they did the right thing, if they understood what was needed or asked for, and if they were generous or withholding. And even if they were basically right, was their behavior impeccable? Over and over, insensitivities, as reported and as manifested in individual and group therapy, are pointed out and examined for the possibility of repair. Patients who have experienced "morally neutral" past therapies may initially be unsettled by this approach.

In cases of exceptional insensitivity, I often seek the help of relationship counselors who are highly adept in spotting and sensitizing individuals to their perceptual and empathetic deficiencies. The first task in these exercises is to get the patient to pay attention to the counselor and to show interest. Then major instances of excessive talking, missing cues, slighting or deflecting remarks, self-preoccupation, and ingratiating over-giving or off-putting holding back are pointed out. A frequent target of attack is the tendency to play favorites among children, colleagues, or employees. In making this mistake, the patient often betrays a major deficit in fairness, which screens out the hurt such favoritism causes to the unfavored. The victims of these hurts, inflicted by parents and grandparents, are certain to keep therapists employed for the foreseeable future.

The meetings with relationship counselors are best held in naturalistic settings such as homes, restaurants, and business offices, where deficient role performance is more readily exposed. It is often astonishing to discover that because of their insensitivity to seemingly obvious cues, these patients have never learned how to behave in public places or in structured dating or interview settings (e.g., berating waiters, using profane language, asking no questions), and these deficiencies in their social skills, which are glaring examples of deficits in human capital, prove to be major obstacles to making their way in life.

3. Channeling and Interiorizing Spiritual Qualities

Developing intrinsic spiritual potential is the highest goal of a spiritual therapy. We all want to strengthen character to the fullest. We want to be able to take principled stands, to do the right thing, and not to be diverted from holding our ground or taking difficult actions because they carry material costs or are met with personal rejection or public opprobrium. And we want to be able to empathize: certainly with those who lay claim to our affections, even when it means overcoming competitive feelings toward them. Among friends, the experience of schadenfreude is certainly the failed litmus test of empathy. But we also want to develop empathy for strangers and foreigners who are going through hard times. Sympathy for their lot and a willingness to work for the alleviation of their suffering are surely the major defining characteristics of that spiritual quality we call being humanitarian.

We note here that developing character is about developing a strong will in the service of promoting enduring values. When our will has been broken because of traumatic past experiences, then character formation necessarily involves the repair of the broken will in all the ways that we have discussed in this book. Integrating split-off partial selves, overcoming the paralysis of depression and the distortions of thought disorder, and taking responsibility and holding others responsible, as opposed to projecting blame or guiltily assuming unwarranted blame—these are some of the steps necessary to strengthening will and forming character.

Becoming empathetic towards others, even when the feeling for them is in the transpersonal mode of *caritas* rather than the personal one of passionate knowing, seems to be more problematic, depending less on hard work than on our innate capacity for sympathy. But just as we can develop character, we can also develop empathy through focus and practice, by paying attention to others and taking the trouble to identify with their experience, by imagining how we would feel if we were in their shoes. Beyond this, we must engage in consciousness-expanding exercises such as meditation, yoga, and the arts, both aesthetic and martial, that induce an awareness (1) that the self is part of a universal Self, in which each of us is a cell in a larger tissue, a small bay of an infinitely large ocean, and (2) that the fate of each is intimately connected to the fate of all; or, as it is often said, "we are all in this together."

But this is not knowledge and virtue that should be paraded before the world. The character and empathy worth their salt are measured by the degree to which they lead to right living and humanitarian contributions, not by the self-importance or acclaim they generate. True spirituality seeks little worldly reward, seeking rather the inner satisfaction of doing the right thing. Therefore, we must not call unnecessary attention to our personal charity but thank the larger Self for making us the instruments of its Will as healers of the sick and poor and finders of the lost. Achieving this focus is what I mean by channeling and interiorizing our spiritual blessings.

Chapter 10
THE CALLING

Summary. Finding one's calling is an essential step in developing a full spiritual life, a necessary prelude to achieving the ultimate state of blessedness. We start from the dictum common to Socratic philosophy and modern psychotherapy: "know thyself." This involves coming to know how we are made, what motivates us, the nature of our skills and talents, and how strongly inspired we are to realize our potential and to make a contribution to the common good. In the process, we recognize our limitations and make corrections when initial plans have proven to be misconceived. Then we must refocus to determine what truly interests us and to determine the means required to turn these interests into a calling that combines self-realization with Self-realization—the union of the individual self's truth with the universal Self's truth. In the process we must develop the strength of character to go beyond convention, faulty conditioning, family disapproval, and even public opprobrium to answer the calling: to express the true self's fundamental longings and the empirical world's greatest needs for healing. The process is guided by an intuitive awareness of universal moral values and critical thinking about the means and consequences of acting on them. The process entails not only strengthening character but also gaining wisdom through education and practical experience in the service of realizing the highest spiritual values.

The idea of a calling or a vocation has its origins in the Torah, where Adam and Eve are called upon in Genesis 2 to "be fertile and increase, fill the earth and master it; and rule the sea, the birds, and the sky, and all living things that creep on earth." The rabbinical commentaries of the Talmud have interpreted this to mean that human beings, made in God's image, are called upon to be godly by becoming creators and acting with love, mercy, and justice; and as their main task, they are "to assist the Creator in perfecting His [imperfect] creation, to become His co-worker" in repairing the world.[87] In the major Christian traditions, the idea of vocation has taken on the more specific meaning of being called to the priesthood in order to elevate humankind from its fallen state by bringing people to believe in Jesus as the

Messiah and to achieve salvation through his love. Christian theology has at times conflated the concept of vocation with notions of predestination and redemption through good works.

In this work I have discussed the elements of a calling in more secular terms: not as a religious mission but as the spiritual ideal of using one's special talents and interests to contribute to the common good. As must be obvious by now, the processes of discovery and execution of the calling are fraught with difficulties. How do we come to know what we are best suited to do? And how do we determine how best to do it to do the most good? The empirical sciences, including the behavioral ones, do not weigh in on these value-laden questions, weighing in only on the means and consequences of taking certain courses of actions rather than others. Psychological insight, in the conventional sense of the product of an applied empirical science, offers little help here, for it is mainly concerned with gaining awareness of one's egocentric needs and conflicts and how to gratify and resolve them to gain the greatest pleasure and the least pain.

A higher order of perception is required to discover who we really are and what really matters. Here we must become aware of what we are specifically and uniquely called to do, to see that it and related activities are the only possible pathways to realizing our potential, which is the main purpose of our lives. I believe that the discovery of individuals' unique missions, what makes their lives worth living, depends on gaining a heightened form of intuitive awareness that transcends empirical and psychological insight to access moral and spiritual truth. This awareness has both an internal and an external aspect. Turned inward, it allows us, often in the wake of powerfully evocative experiences, to come to know the true self and its basic intentions and values and more specifically to hear clearly and persuasively the promptings of conscience. Turned outward, it informs us of who and what manifests great moral wisdom and power and how we can contribute to their deployment for healing the maladies of the empirical world.

Exercising a calling is joyous work. In fact it is more like play. We typically become absorbed in doing it without much self-doubt and even less self-consciousness. We look forward to doing it because it feels continually rewarding and seems to flow naturally from our strongest interests and talents while giving the satisfaction of being worthwhile and meaningful. Rather than the drudgery of work-work, it affords the pleasure of play-work.

"Play" may have for some the wrong connotation. But for those fortunate enough to answer a calling, working at it at least feels like *significant* play, in the sense that it is absorbing, fulfilling, and a source of joy. Those who have found a calling inevitably say that it gives great meaning to their lives. In fact, a strong case can be made that finding and pursuing a vocation is one of the two main reasons we find ourselves as conscious beings on this planet in the cosmos. The other is to find loved ones who join with us in the awe of mutual love and the thrill of mutual creation: children, of course, but also projects, inventions, and causes. In the process the individual self becomes one with the universal Self. In sum, we know that we have found a calling when these conditions are met: we feel strongly impelled to do the work, it gives full creative expression to our true self's best talents and qualities, and it affords us the satisfaction of contributing to the common good by working in synergy with others. At best there is congruence between what we uniquely have to offer and what makes the world a better place.

"The Lord's Work"

I doubt that finding a calling on these terms is commonplace. In our fast-moving society disoriented by a cultural revolution that calls into question all spiritual values, distractions all too easily drown out the call from the true self and its guiding spirit to do what we are put here to do. Perceiving few practical alternatives, we often settle for making a good living in comfortable circumstances. We have stopped worrying about whether we have fully realized our potential and used our skills and talents to "repair the world." Instead we are satisfied to follow in the footsteps of parents or teachers or to go where the pay is high and the hours are short. We might be aware that something is missing, but we are not motivated to find out what that something is.

By way of contrast, the spiritually inclined cannot comfortably settle for an ordinary job, much less an ordinary life. Those of us who aspire to attaining spiritual consciousness cannot be content until we have found a *lifework*: a highly meaningful activity that draws on our best to do our best. Consider these two contrasting examples.

Mr. J was highly animated as he described the vagaries of his work in the sale of commodities. A few days earlier, he had urgently flown from Newark to Bangkok because a customer would not pay the agreed-upon price for a shipment. The customer claimed that the product did not meet the specifications of the original contract. In fact, the market price for this commodity had dropped significantly since the customer signed the order, and he was obviously trying to improve the terms of his mistimed purchase. Mr. J clearly relished recounting the charade of haggling, dining, and drinking that followed in an effort to close the deal. I remarked that he seemed to derive great enjoyment out of this kind of combat, to which he replied, "Well, it's not the Lord's work, but it sure is interesting."

Sandy, the middle-aged woman we first met in chapter 2, was a writer and corporate trainer. Although extremely bright and talented, she had never found work that satisfied her. She had run a restaurant, taught writing and literature in high schools and colleges, and finally had high-paying jobs in corporate training, from the last of which she had been recently fired. She felt no sense of fulfillment or meaning in any of these misadventures. In a new corporate training job after starting treatment, she found her calling by transforming ordinary coaching into mentoring in which she used her caring, empathetic personality to help her trainees come alive and gain confidence in their competence and purpose, as a good parental role model typically does. The model for this transformation came from her work with a depressed fellow group member, Johanna, who claimed that Sandy breathed life into her. The group also dissuaded her from reaping the conventional benefits of her newfound success: a promotion up the corporate hierarchy. Such promotions often move a person from a joyful calling into a more routine bureaucratic post, where meaningful work on the front lines of need and deed is traded for the barren hills of higher pay and administrative authority.

Mr. J had no conscious interest in what I am calling a calling. Yet he was very successful and enjoyed no lack of satisfaction at work. A very decent man, he was mainly concerned with having honest work for which he was well paid and appreciated. He had good values. Not materialistic or ostentatious, he treasured his family and friends, advocated for progressive political causes, and thoroughly enjoyed movies and plays. We might conclude that he had no spiritual interests, but this would be a mistake. Being honest and loyal and caring toward family, friends, and the state of society are surely manifestations of spiritual values. The fact that he knew his work was not "the Lord's work" is also a tip-off that he had intimations of the qualities of living a calling. Yet consciously seeking one would, I am certain, feel pretentious to him, just as making any claim that he was doing "the Lord's work" would feel immodest and self-serving. As in the case of the previously mentioned owners of the inn in France who hid local Jews from Nazi roundups, being loyal to family and friends and making common cause and showing common decency count toward spirituality whether or not there is a conscious sense of it. We should not let our consideration of ideal forms of spirituality blind us to its everyday manifestations. The ideal ought never to become the enemy of the real.

Obstacles

The obstacles lying in the path of finding a vocation are everywhere. Sometimes neither the material resources nor the opportunities are readily available. When certain pursuits are mentioned, well-intentioned colleagues or family members argue fiercely against their feasibility, undermining an already shaky resolve. A significant number of my patients, to their later regret, have been pushed into professional work by parents who thought it impractical for them to pursue a career in writing or playing an instrument. As if parental disapproval were not daunting enough, some have suffered devastating psychological and physical traumas early in life, like the loss of a limb or a beloved parent, that virtually extinguished the creative spark and left them with constricted expectations of themselves and of life in general; they often curdle with bitterness toward an unjust world. Major acts of will are required to rise above these catastrophic losses to regain the creative, healing aspirations of a spiritual life. Instead those whose spiritual fires have been banked settle for jobs or professions that do not realize their potential or satisfy their hunger for meaningful purpose. Even when these obstacles have been overcome, not everyone has the discipline to devote the more than 10,000 hours of practice—Malcolm Gladwell's number—required to develop effective expertise in a serious pursuit.[88]

Victims of Success

Another major clinical problem arises when people choose security over spirituality even when they have strong spiritual potential. For example, Mr. Davis, the CEO of a large insurance company, constantly obsessed about his board's disapproval, the value of his perks, and his wife's complaints about his emotional unavailability. His job felt like a prison sentence rather than a rewarding achievement. His overbearing mother had groomed him to be the corporate success that she, as a traditional woman of her time, had been denied. But with each move up the corporate ladder, he felt more isolated and less fulfilled. Every time he was on the brink of breaking out of this vicious cycle by doing something connected with his interest in the arts or a philanthropic venture, some new award that claimed more of his time was foisted upon him. He felt victimized by his success. For lack of courage or sense of higher purpose, Mr. Davis could never bring himself to turn down a promotion and its expanded responsibilities in order to do what he loved.

At the time of our work together, I had not yet developed the approach, dependent in part on strong group support, to help rescue him from this impasse. But his situation forced me to reckon with the extreme difficulty of renouncing power, status, and money to pursue something as insubstantial as an ideal. Those who have the strong character to do it without a strong support system tailored to bolster the effort are deserving of great admiration, more so if they can transform their work into a lifework of creative, healing expression. Given good leadership, imagine what a large insurance company might do in the aftermath of devastations such as Hurricane Katrina or Sandy to promote the building of flood-protected housing in places such as New Orleans's Ward 9, as individuals such as Vinod Khosla, cofounder of Sun Microsystems, have successfully done.

Overcoming the Obstacles

An effective spiritual group therapy holds promise of helping those who cannot on their own abandon an unfulfilling line of work to find their calling. It can provide both the opportunity and the methodology. A successful outcome depends on realizing all the components of the approach that we have so far discussed. Individuals must locate their true self—what their real interests, talents, and values are—and then allow themselves to be influenced by their guiding spirit to discard the unfulfilling goals pursued by their false self. This process is often abetted by exploring the origins of the false self in the traumas and empathic failures of past experience. As for Mr. Davis, his mother foisted her own ambitions on him without the empathy and respect for autonomy to let him determine his own interests and goals. This misdirection was clearly a determining factor in his unhappy life and called for a probing understanding of the causative role it played. Achievement of such understanding is typically followed by a reformulation of the goals of the persons' real versus fase selves. Then such individuals have to develop the strength of character to make a break with their past histories and, if need be, certain ocupations and relationships, to develop their true purpose. Typically, they must also find influential mentors who can give the necessary social support essential to taking these painful steps.

Mr. Davis needed strong guidance and support to jump off the treadmill of success and failure as defined by his mother, wife, and corporate board, to seek out those activities that accorded with his inner nature. Often this is an ideal time to retire "for reasons of health and family" from one's day job. This excuse is not entirely misleading once we recognize that true and full health must include working toward the achievement of spiritual ideals, not only for the best health of the individual but also for that of family and ever larger circles of friends and fellow human beings.

A spiritual group can give the support and collective wisdom to make the necessary changes: to affirm one's true self, to discern and act on the confluence of one's talents, interests, and social needs that would turn a career into a calling. Perhaps Mr. Davis could have used his executive skills to direct an arts program or, as indicated, even to change part of the mission of his insurance company to better support recovery from the ever more frequent disasters of our climate-changing and globalizing world.

Implications

There are several implications of this discussion. One is that you do not always have to leave your current work to find a vocation, but you may have to change some part of it to make it vocation-worthy, to make it expressive of your best talents while being socially reparative. But not every line of work is susceptible to this kind of transformation, in which case you must either take leave of it or stay forever locked into its limitations. There is no way to salvage a job in sales and turn it into a calling if the marketed products are dangerous or worthless. You will have to find better products or a line of work that is more expressive of your better self. Unfortunately, as with bad marriages, we cannot usually leave even unfulfilling work unless the high costs of staying and the existence of alternative paths and the means to follow them are made painfully evident. Not making changes in these circumstances is eerily reminiscent of the case of the individual who gambled with his health by refusing to take his anti-diabetes medicine, with blindness, circulatory failure, and premature death destined to follow.

Ruined health and ruined life are the inevitable consequences of remaining in soul-destroying situations. *Destrudo*, the self-destructive "instinct," can take many forms, and its existence poses the most severe challenges to those who wish to rewrite their destinies.

Spiritual Groups and False Paths

A spiritual group and its leader, with their power to deploy strong incentives and disincentives, can make life-changing contributions to individuals enmeshed in these wrong-path situations. Effective spiritual groups provide inspiring examples of individuals, such as Sandy and Sarah, the failed jazz singer, who have left or transformed unfulfilling lines of work to find their calling. Pointing the way, various members also model the kinds of effort required to make the necessary changes. They show how the anxieties and insecurities of a life-altering transition can be managed. And they provide examples of "reading the tea leaves," of recognizing which types of work might be worthy and feasible as vocations for particular individuals with unique needs and abilities. At its best, the spiritual group is ideally constructed to offer powerful feedback and supportive pressure to launch the seeker onto the pathways of spiritual transformation. Such changes are not for the faint of heart, nor can they usually be accomplished by the solitary adventurer, cut off from a knowledgeable, caring support system that includes a mentoring role model.

The Mission and the Enablers

I believe that each of us comes into adulthood with a particular life mission and that it is our highest obligation to overcome all obstacles to finding it and carrying it out. Some of us are meant to serve others diligently and faithfully, whether in a high or a low capacity. I doubt that many of us would be where we are today were it not for the love and guidance shown us as children by teachers, coaches, and leaders, alongside emotionally and intellectually available parents or guardians. Some of us are inclined to be teachers or healers, an intentionality that inspirational school or college teachers and, later, therapists augmented by opening our eyes to the love of knowledge and insight and the aesthetic experience of truth and beauty. Such teachers do this not only by formal teaching but also through the example of their own love of knowledge and truth and their interest in us as people. Craftspeople, teachers, inventors, performers, artists, soldiers, statesmen, coaches, seekers of truth, healers, pioneers, scourges—each of us is made to join the ranks of one or more of these vocations. And find the right ones we must! But events and early conditioning can conspire to send us off on paths of regret.

Retracing our steps and finding the right path is often a perilous undertaking. Access may be extremely difficult. The obstacles we have already mentioned often come into play. And the appropriate line of work may be hidden in a buzzing, blooming confusion of choices of seemingly equal value, further obscured by well-intentioned bad advice from family and friends. After taking the wrong paths, we find ourselves years later practicing law or medicine or working for a corporation, hating every minute of it and maybe not doing a great job either, because it's work-work, not play-work. It has become sterile and onerous, not expressive of our true talents and values and therefore not done in a way that generates the love that comes from strengthening our character and repairing the world. Taking many small steps toward repairing will and world is the ultimate purpose and inevitable outcome of answering the call with passion and good faith.

The Clues

What are the clues to recognizing a potential calling? Certainly luck and blink[89] often play a part. Opportunities crop up and smack us in the face, and sparked with enthusiasm, we run with them down the path to fulfillment. But it is not always so easy. Many patients come to therapy after years of struggle without ever finding work that clicks. The first thing we have to consider is that they are already in a position to find it, but their emotional headwinds and cognitive boxes pose insuperable obstacles. Maybe they are too depressed or cognitively disordered to recognize the opportunities that lie at hand. The usual issues must be addressed: untreated depression, confusion, harsh conscience, and parental injunctions, all amenable to improvement by modern psychiatric treatment. I am often amazed at how quickly patients find their path once depression is resolved, sometimes through therapy alone, sometimes through a combination of therapy and medicine.

Ben, a thirty-four-year-old single man, adrift and plagued by anxiety and low self-esteem, had neither meaningful work nor a romantic relationship. For many years he had languished in a dead-end job as a social worker at a poorly run agency. His mother's lifelong worries about his emotional frailty and inability to succeed on the level of his high school classmates conveyed a general lack of appreciation of his virtues. He heard over and over in his head his mother's constant lament: "Poor Ben! Poor Ben!"

Actually, the main poor thing about him was the burden of carrying his mother's projections and their harmful effects on his mood and self-confidence. He was intrinsically a very caring person with altruistic values. And he had years of practice absorbing his mother's distress without losing his core strength and integrity.

After undergoing appropriate medical and psychological treatment and briefly cutting off contact with his intrusive, enveloping mother, he soon discovered that he was romantically attracted to his best friend at work, a woman who had been patiently waiting for him to notice her affection for him. They would soon marry and start a family. With renewed confidence, he applied for a job at a renowned pediatric hospital. Down the road, he became head family counselor at the hospital. He continues to do grief counseling with the parents of children suffering from cancer and severe chronic illnesses, work that is less difficult for him than for most caregivers. As someone whose mother frequently voiced fears of dying from cancer as he grew up, he learned over the years how to cushion these burdens without losing his capacity for empathy, without losing his soul. Painful as the work still proves to be, he feels every day that he is making a critical difference in the ability of these children and their families to cope with their tragedies. He and his wife volunteer every summer as counselors at a camp for these chronically ill children.

His new sense of fulfillment both at home and at work is reflected in his body language and his verbal language. He shows pride in himself and his life. His mother was right, though: in material terms, he has not succeeded at the level of some of his high school and college classmates, especially those who manage large corporations or hedge funds. Unlike them, he has no golden parachute to mitigate the damage to his own and his clients' assets when economic and emotional bubbles burst. Make no mistake—he is prone to a sense of failure every time one of his patients dies or suffers relapse. Yet he manages these failures by realizing that he has done his best to help them: he has modeled coping methods and given comfort to these patients and their families through their crises. There are no lasting failures when one is living a calling, only misconceived past expectations, remedied by reconceiving them as opportunities for future learning and healing.

Going Farther Afield

As we have suggested, sometimes patients have to go farther afield to find their calling because their original choice of profession proves to be too contaminated with false values or too alien to their core interests to yield a promising line of work. In these cases, we must be on the lookout for clues as to what activities, perhaps in their nonwork lives, engage their passions. Sometimes it is political action in the service of a cause, such as promoting energy conservation, aiding the victims of persecution around the world, or tending to those afflicted with some dreaded disease such as AIDS or leukemia. To be engaged with the requisite passion to pursue these causes in a vocational mode, it helps if there is some personal connection, such as a loved relative or friend who has suffered or died from the condition. The possibility of finding a vocation is also greatly enhanced if the new career does not go *too far* afield from the individual's basic training. For instance, a patient who did not enjoy the practice of commercial law felt a much greater sense of mission when he became an advocate for public-sector rehabilitation programs for addicts. And a nurse who worked for charitable organizations before nursing training was disgusted with all the backbiting and petty stresses of hospital practice. But once she took the opportunity to do inoculations and infectious disease control in impoverished Latin American villages, she felt that this public health work was both rewarding and meaningful.

Of course, these vocational ventures might seem relatively easy to undertake if we have a large nest egg to offset the financial drag of a career change. But even absent significant wealth, how much real sacrifice is entailed when, in a society such as ours, we can forego purchasing an expensive automobile for an inexpensive one, and we can stop eating at highly rated restaurants in favor of home-cooking or good ethnic eateries, without making significant compromises in quality of life? To be sure, some compromises in comforts and luxuries may have to be made. But we are speaking of finding a calling—a lifework!—in place of a job, and we have to affirm the values and make the commitments to bring it about. No one can convince us it is worth the sacrifices entailed unless we can afford to make them—financially, emotionally, and spiritually.

Charitable Giving versus Practicing a Calling

Once we focus on the values and commitments at issue, we quickly realize that philanthropic giving alone may not qualify as a calling. Hands-on involvement with the process and the beneficiaries of our charity may also be required to give the giving a sense of worth and fulfillment. We cannot expect to pull people out of the mud without getting our hands dirty. So it is one thing to give money to organizations that promote AIDS treatment in Africa or music education in the schools and quite another also to have direct involvement: to go to the clinics and schools, to give organizational support on-site, to find and subsidize worthy experts and appropriate role models to make an impact, and to help to secure the training of those experts and models so that they can do a better job of treating and teaching. Only then would we go beyond ordinary philanthropy, a distant support of causes, to having a vocation in education or relief of poverty and disease.

Beyond its great recruitment methods and outstanding faculty, one of the reasons the Curtis Institute of Music is such a preeminent conservatory for the education of young musicians is the fact that many of its charitable donors also serve as substitute parents for these young prodigies, who are often living and studying in Philadelphia while their families remain behind in China or Uzbekistan. Their new adoptive families feed them, host practice concerts, drive them to doctors, and support them through homesickness and lovesickness—all in addition to contributing money to the institution. This may not be on the scale of Bill Gates's calling as a donor to education and health development, but these "little" contributions by everyday people add up to a mighty force for good.

The Truth about Ourselves

Many of the obstacles to finding a calling have already been mentioned. The inertia that blocks change is always a major difficulty. This is especially the case when, as with Mr. Davis, there are financial and emotional rewards for staying put and great sacrifices for pursuing a dream. And there may be clinical obstacles: depression, confused thinking, inhibitions, materialistic indoctrination, emotional deprivations, and narcissistic injuries—the list of biological and psychological impediments to pursuing a spiritual vocation is long. As mentioned, friends and colleagues, mired in their own routines, may also become envious, even feel reproached by our idealistic plans, and feel constrained to discourage us from such impractical ventures.

There are purely spiritual obstacles as well. It is not just that some individuals have little spiritual potential. It is also that there are dangers to pursuing a life of spiritual meaning, and perceiving these dangers leads to legitimate apprehensions. The hard truth is that no matter how noble the aspirations, many career changes fail to meet expectations. Think of all the great cooks who don't make a go of it as restaurant owners and all the fine teachers who undertake progressive modes of education that ultimately bear little fruit. In some cases, the fervor of the ideals is not matched by a mastery of the marketing and management skills crucial to success in practice. In other cases, spiritual passion crosses over into grandiosity, and the mission, so sound on paper, turns into a self-righteous authoritarian nightmare. The fallout from Bruno Bettelheim's Orthogenic School[90] in Chicago is still being felt in some circles, and only a few generations ago, the casualties of Gurdjieff's[91] spiritual mentoring were still washing up on the shores of Europe and America.

This brings us to perhaps the greatest obstacle of all: the difficulty of accepting the truth about ourselves. What can I possibly mean? Put simply, we all have serious limitations. Even though we may have insights into infinite truth, we are ourselves finite. If we forget this, we may overvalue what lies in the core of our being and formulate a mission that is too grand for our modest talents. We may not be organized well enough or have the leadership abilities or the sheer drive to accomplish the mission as initially envisioned. This is where a spiritual group and its leader have crucial information to convey. The truth must be told and accepted. Sandy needed to be told that her original aspirations for great success in the corporate world were misplaced, as were her aspirations to be a public poet. Even though she had enjoyed past successes in both fields, they were not sustainable. And the reasons were obvious to her therapist and her group. She was, at the very least, not disciplined enough to get the job done. Successful writers write every day on a fairly regular schedule, and no matter how many letters of rejection they receive, they continue to submit their work and to maintain connections with people in the field. She did none of these things in a sustained way. Those who are successful in corporate life must be capable of working cooperatively, must get their work done on time, and must be able to understand the corporate task and to operate within its structure. Sandy, again, prior to treatment, could not do these things on a consistent basis. All her successes were based on generic competence and, more fundamentally, the warmth and dynamism of her personality. Therefore, any line of work that she could be successful at would most likely depend on these attributes as the central driving force. This means that the work would essentially involve maintaining personal interfaces. The counseling-coaching-therapy interface would be an ideal locus, provided that she could bring her formal organizational and teaching skills up to a consistently professional level to maintain a midlevel executive position. Without sacrificing a newfound sense of calling in the work, this she was ultimately able to do.

Similarly, it was difficult for the already mentioned graduate of Harvard's law and business schools to accept that he did not have the leadership and management skills to run a corporation. Those deficits were crucial reasons that employees did not respect or fear his authority enough to desist from stealing hundreds of thousands of dollars of inventory. It was apparent that he was a brilliant man but more of a retiring intellectual than a leader. He would have done better to follow a career in education or something in the nonprofit sphere rather than one in the highly competitive world of business and manufacture. His problem with accepting this verdict, and also the evidence for its truth, became clear at the first marital conference. His wife was the dominant force in the marriage, and she insisted that he run a big corporation as a symbol of her own status in the world. Like certain political marriages, he was to be the spear carrier of her ambitions, but the spear he wielded was made of too malleable a substance.

A different twist on the acceptance theme concerned the truth about Carl, already discussed in a prior chapter. His father, who had been an expert in financial manipulations, got caught defrauding investors and either committed suicide or was the victim of a mob hit when Carl was ten. To avoid the shame, Carl's mother, who was implicated in the tragedy by the way she had pushed her husband to make more and more money, moved the family out of the country for the next several years. In addition to the devastation of losing his father and the attendant neurotic guilt, Carl also suffered the added trauma of losing his friends and teachers and having to adapt to a hostile new environment, all at the beginning of puberty. In treatment he was able to overcome his suicidal impulses, get married, start a family, and develop a business that felt worthwhile. Securing a major market share for home health care workers, he made a good living while feeling proud that he was performing a service to the community.

But in the first flush of success, he overexpanded. He began to buy pieces of real estate, and he bowed to his wife's insistence on having one child after another, even though they both came from families with histories of severe mental illness. As might be expected, four of their five children had major behavioral problems, and the bills for treatment and special schools were astronomical. And several of the real estate investments didn't pan out. Carl began to feel a cash-flow crunch that kept him up at night.

The whole edifice began to crumble when his wife became angrily paranoid and relentlessly blamed Carl for everything that was wrong with her life: their disturbed children, her domestic burdens, problems with their large home with a leaky roof, and his emotional withdrawal. Unable to defend himself against this onslaught, he quietly absorbed her anger and crumbled inside, developing a major depressive episode. He became paralyzed in his ability to make timely decisions. When she refused to relent, he could not get out of the line of fire by moving out. Symbolic of his dysfunction, he could not make the decisions to get the house's leaky roof repaired. No amount of group support or medication changes allayed his anxiety and sense of having a leaky roof himself. With Carl now posing a serious suicidal risk, a joint family conference was set up with his wife and her therapist, in which everyone came to the agreement that they could avoid hospitalization for Carl only by calling a truce to the angry complaining and blaming, which his wife, with her therapist's support, was able to honor enough to make a difference.

In this less hostile environment and after selling off some of his holdings, Carl slowly reorganized and was able to put his main business back on a solid basis. And if his wife slipped, he was able to ask her to hold off from yelling at him because it was making him sick. But the truth about himself was a bitter pill to swallow. Like his father he was basically defenseless, initially lacking the kind of character strength that would protect him from being knocked off-course if he were pushed hard. He had to accept that without calling in outside help, he could neither contain his wife's fury nor prevent her from driving him crazy. Carl lacked the strength to put his foot down, which, paradoxically, always comes down to showing a willingness to end the relationship in the absence of required changes. That we have certain faults in our character strength is one of the most disturbing facts we as human beings have to recognize about ourselves, but admitting this is far more courageous than denying the truth, and it opens up the possibility of reaching out for the help we need to start the process of becoming strong and judicious enough to erect defenses, typically with the help of others.

After he fully recognized his weakness, Carl did become strong enough to tell his wife the truth about his eroded love for her and to move toward divorce.

His improvement involved not only getting separated but also accepting the painful fact that, as with many who lose a parent during certain crucial early developmental stages, he could not defend himself out of fear that any show of aggression was tantamount to killing his adversary. He remembers hearing the news of his father's death while at camp. Before that time, he had been a good athlete and eager to go out each day to hit the ball. After his father's death, he abruptly lost athletic ability and all other competencies that required competitive aggression.

Recapitulation

The spiritual therapy that we have explored in this book relies on the whole armamentarium of modern psychiatry: psychoactive medication, cognitive relearning, psychodynamic understanding, family and group restructuring, and above all spiritual group therapy. All teachers of the spiritual life start with the command "Attention! Attention!" Pay attention to the details; develop the discipline to adhere to the rules and observe the boundaries, breaking them only with careful compensation; and above all, learn to oscillate between the spiritual and the sensible, the calling and the answering. There is no calling worth its name that does not answer to the needs and the welfare of those whom we serve.

All of these treatment modalities are deployed to free the will, clarify thinking, enhance knowledge, strengthen character, deepen empathy, acknowledge limitations, live with dignity, and find a calling. In the process, we realize the wisdom of the ages:

Know your conscious, unconscious, and true spiritual self.

Honor your true self and its ideals by following its guiding spirit.

Do not hide behind the will of others.

Take responsibility for all your actions.

Recognize that we are often bringing about what seems to be happening to us.

Fight for integrity because the dissociated self cannot realize its full potential.

Treat all people as ends in themselves and as you would have them treat you.

Free the will by overcoming inborn and learned deficits and inhibitions.

Develop character by repeated acts of will.

Accept the truth about limitations and thereby gain the freedom to grow stronger.

Do "the Lord's work"—that is, promote the well-being of all.

Make common cause with like-minded souls. The will of the people united is a mighty force.

Chapter 11
BLESSEDNESS

Summary. The manifest feeling states of achieving blessedness are joy and fullness. Joy, not mere pleasure or happiness, is the glory of having achieved spiritual consciousness with its attendant sense of consonance with the universal love and will of Spirit. There is no greater sense of fulfillment than being filled with Spirit. We are truly blessed to achieve this state, for we are thereby given the capacity to give and receive love, to intuit the moral law, to see the splendor and order of nature, to feel a sense of belonging to family, society, and cosmos; and we are given the will to find our calling and the character strength to overcome all obstacles to its achievement. What joy to know that we share in one all-embracing consciousness, the transcendent Self, in whose participation we join all conscious beings!

The ultimate purpose of a spiritual therapy is to achieve a state of blessedness—blessedness rather than happiness because blessedness cannot be mistaken for anything less than a profound state of spiritual joy. In contrast, happiness may be defined by states of ordinary well-being that do not attach enduringly to the true self and its connection to Spirit. This is not to say that feeling happy and content cannot be a vitally important constituent and outward sign of blessedness but to say that the core state goes beyond any ordinary satisfactions and sense of achievement to give vivid testimony that the blessed person is a spiritual person in harmony with the universe. The Sufi saints have called this state "the great peace."

In the course of the discussion that follows, we must not forget that this harmony will forever elude us if we do not accept that we are living in the sensible world on borrowed time. In this world, the cycles of living and dying are of the essence, and this essential truth applies to all living beings. Since we cannot escape this fate, the sense of blessedness crucially depends on our making peace with our biological mortality.[92] It is our great good fortune that the spiritual Self lies outside time and its cycles of birth and decay, so that in a sense what will be has always been. We are blessed to achieve communion with this timeless aspect of life.

In the short term, those who feel blessed typically enjoy reasonably good health. At the very least, they are not suffering unbearable pain, and their quality of life has not been so diminished that they cannot enjoy being alive. But what we might call good health is by no means essential. We have all met individuals of great fortitude whose suffering partakes of the sacred. Severely limited and in pain from the effects of a crippling accident or progressive illness, they nevertheless feel blessed right up to their last, agonized breath. This was clearly true of an acquaintance, progressively paralyzed by multiple sclerosis, who pointed to her unwavering gratitude for her life and its relative impermeability to the ravages of loss with the title of her memoir, *You Are Not Your Illness*.[93] How could one not be inspired by the courage of a friend who maintained a positive attitude and even her exercise routine despite crippling pain from metastatic cancer until the day before she died? At the end, as she took her final breaths, she spoke to her husband of gratitude for her life and for her dreams of a peaceful world.

Such phenomena shed light on two related aspects of blessedness. First, blessed individuals have the strength of character to compartmentalize pain and suffering in order to retain a spiritual self that lies outside the daily battering of the conscious, empirical self and, more profoundly, to regard the inevitable failures that punctuate our successes as establishing the inextricability of good and ill, joy and suffering, material losses and spiritual gains in the course of all human life.

Second, those who feel blessed have a belief system powerful enough to allow them to compartmentalize, to dissociate in the service of health. Such a belief system typically teaches us to focus on the positive aspects of life, to regard all negative feelings and experiences as situations calling for remedial action or, failing that, as occasions to accept the workings of a higher purposeful order that we call fate, the life force, or Spirit. The articles of our faith accomplish this by urging us to give more weight to gratitude for experiences of love, goodness, and truth than to hate, evil, and falsehood in whatever forms they take. We avoid negativity in our thinking and in the people and causes with which we choose to associate. We try our best not to succumb to resentment for the crippling of our bodies, the demise of loved ones, and the decline of cherished abilities and stature, all inevitably associated with the life-and-death cycle of mortal beings.

Love Partners

The blessed person gives and receives love. Our first experiences of love usually involve our parents and siblings. Later, if we are very fortunate, we fall in love with that special person who becomes our soul mate as we achieve physical and spiritual union. We know we are on the right track when, from the very beginning, we enjoy being with the other person and laugh together at what we both recognize as inevitable, absurd, and uncanny. Over time, the other person's happiness makes us happy, and his or her sadness makes us sad; we take pleasure in our mate's pleasure and feel pain when he or she is in pain. Envy and resentment have no permanent place in these unions because our souls have joined together to make common cause. We come to share in each other's satisfactions and miseries, and we accord each other infinite, irreplaceable value. This kind of love, embracing the continuum of physical and spiritual union, may be our first intimation of the existence of a higher consciousness, an encompassing, permeating Spirit constituted, at least in part, by the union of individual minds.

The Platonic Spiritual Love of Individuals and Groups

A purely spiritual love, shorn of its physical dimension, may attach to very close friends and also to leaders and followers and teachers and students who have a mentoring relationship. To qualify as mentoring, the learning process must involve not just the attainment of special skills but also guided development of aesthetic, moral, and spiritual values taught in the context of a caring relationship. Our most influential teachers and guides manifest a selfless regard for our growth and welfare that goes beyond any specific subject matter to point the way to leading a meaningful and beneficent life, filled with appreciation and wonderment. In return we feel reverence and gratitude for their caring generosity. It should go without saying that there can be no spiritual therapy, as we have defined it, unless these conditions are met in the relationship between therapists and patients.

Spiritual love may also exist between the members of a group. In previous chapters, I have described many of the preconditions for the formation of a spiritual group. The membership must be restricted to potentially spiritual individuals. This means they must all have an intact conscience, an intrinsic sense of right and wrong, and the ability to transcend selfish needs to care about each other. Antisocial, paranoid, and addicted individuals, for obvious reasons, do not pass these tests. Less obviously, those who are highly competitive and jealous have great difficulty in recognizing the merits of colleagues, who are always seen as potential rivals. Colleagues' successes and failures, instead of inspiring admiration and sympathetic support, become occasions for reevaluating competitive rankings. In contrast, colleagues who are spiritually connected do not feel schadenfreude (or if so, only transiently) when their fellow members experience failure and loss.

Other kinds of groups characterized by spiritual caring may include athletic teams engaged in the common pursuit of playing their best to win. The condition may be met when the manager or coach has inspirational leadership qualities and the resultant heightened ability to get initially egocentric players to become team players and, if that proves impossible, to cut them out of the mix. The qualities of spiritual connection are likely to be even more pronounced in a group devoted to a noble cause, such as combating disease and poverty, providing big brothers and sisters or parental surrogates to broken families, fostering the education of the underprivileged, and providing aid to the victims of war, natural disasters, and plagues. A community of adherents to a philosophic or religious belief system has its greatest impact when the members achieve mutual caring in their devotion to realizing their common goals. The sense of spiritual value that derives from these memberships accords closely with the sense of shared mission that arises from the spiritual therapy group work that I have described in earlier chapters. In fact, the spiritual group, intrinsic to our approach to therapy, provides a template for patients as they seek to duplicate its sense of meaningful participation in their lives outside of treatment.

Most importantly, what I discovered early in my career was that under special circumstances the patients and staff of a mental hospital can be joined together in a common spiritual dedication to the pursuit of mental health. The requisite developmental sequence can then be exported into the outpatient setting, the achievement of which has been a main focus of this book.

Whether or not one has a special love-partner or soul mate, I do not believe that blessedness comes easily to those who do not go beyond dyadic relationships to participate in spiritual groups. In the Judaic and Christian traditions, and also in our legacy from Greek culture and the Enlightenment, the main sources of our Western worldview, we pursue the spiritual life in everyday affairs, not in isolated, otherworldly retreats, as in some Eastern belief systems. Despite the distractions afforded by the "buzzing, blooming confusion" of the marketplace and the playground, following the spiritual path in the world's rough-and-tumble has the singular advantage of throwing us into relationships with a vast range of personalities, events, and challenges that help us locate and develop our true and unique self. In this way, we realize its manifold potentialities. As George Herbert Mead pointed out, our sense of self is defined, at least in part, in its relationship to "the generalized other," the abstracted common qualities, good and bad, of all the people we interact with.[94] Only by virtue of these interactions do we come to fully know ourselves in both our sacred and our profane aspects.

Love and the Creation or Destruction of Spirit

Loving and being loved by another is the usual portal of entry into the spiritual life because spirit is often first experienced when two souls unite, the union with a loving mother serving as the ideal model for later adult unions outside the family. The mini-spirit generated by two adults in spiritual union, facilitated by physical union, is the common creation of all couples truly and deeply in love. The implication of our discussion, however, is that participating in Spirit in its largest and most inclusive sense—becoming part of the world spirit or life force, or in religious parlance standing naked and open before the divine presence—involves the psychic union of ever larger groups of minds. The magnetic, adhesive force that brings this about is nothing other than spiritual love. What we know for certain is that being unable to love is to be damned to never feeling blessed.

In Dostoyevsky's masterpiece, *The Brothers Karamazov*, the great teacher, Father Zossima, makes one of the most singularly important statements in all literature: "Fathers and teachers, I ponder, 'What is hell?' I maintain it is the suffering of being unable to love." The truth of Zossima's declaration is amply borne out by patients who, having fallen into a state of melancholic depression, discover that they no longer have any feelings of affection at all, even for their previously beloved children, whose adorable qualities are no longer experienced as having emotional depth. This is universally described as a state of living hell. Without the capacity to love, to have caring affection, one can neither inspire love nor experience the giving or receiving of it. One has lost one's soul.

Family Belonging, Adoption, and the Special Importance of Grandchildren

When our love extends beyond a love partner to loyal friends, to parents and grandparents, and especially to children and grandchildren, new vistas of blessedness open up to us. The glory of fathering and mothering, of having progeny who are themselves miracles of creation and who visibly serve as channels for the transmission of both our genetic inheritance and our unique familial spirit, is certainly one of the peak experiences of any life. Conversely, any obstacle to assuming one's rightful place in this chain of being, any thwarting of membership in one's rightful lineage, constitutes the most important source of the kinds of emotional deficits that erect impenetrable barriers to achieving the blessed state. We see this clearly in some patients who were put up for adoption as infants and whose adoptive parents lack the fundamentals of caring warmth. They have suffered not only a personal abandonment, but also a severing of the enlivening roots of their inheritance, of the nourishment derived from connecting to an ancestral family spirit or even a transplanted one. When adoption may be the least bad choice, as when children are placed with competent, caring adoptive parents because biological parents are unable or unwilling, the children, in the absence of extraordinary compensatory attention, all too often manifest post-traumatic as well as depressive and physical symptoms. These include a nameless sense of loss, an inability ever to feel fully satisfied, a core anxious inadequacy, a panic-stricken reaction to even minor separations, and a host of what are loosely called psychosomatic disorders, typically affecting the gastrointestinal, immune, and circulatory systems. Such symptoms may contaminate the individual's entire life experience. As indicated, the beginnings of repair may come with getting married and having children, especially if one succeeds in overcoming the damage to the capacity to bond with others through a steady, relentless nurturance from a new family whose love cannot be denied.

Sometimes the damage is manifested in the workings of a split-off saboteur, described earlier, that reenacts the early traumatic abandonment in relationships to children and prospective lovers. For example, one adoptee patient could not bear to be alone with her newborn infant, whom she repeatedly handed off to nurses before bolting from the room in a state of panic. A review of her adoptive history and a barrage of supportive interpretations and limit-setting on her acting out were essential to her stopping the panicky behavior pattern. But such interventions may not be nearly as effective as the mere fact of having grandchildren. Beyond the most powerful forms of psychotherapy, having grandchildren gives birth to a new spiritual lifeline that replaces the previously severed connections of parental and family loss, seen most dramatically in early abandonments.

In a case previously discussed, Paula was given away at six months of age to an adoptive mother who soon became chronically bedridden with a progressive illness. Later, suffering from depression and a severe autoimmune disease, Paula searched out her biological mother, only to discover that she was intermittently psychotic and had given birth to and given away other children as well. The birth mother's unresponsiveness to Paula made her feel traumatically rejected all over again, precipitating an exacerbation of symptoms. Later, with good medical management, her autoimmune disorder went into remission. But depression remained partially refractory to the most broad-gauged biological, psychological, and spiritual therapy that my team and I could offer. Only with the birth of her grandchildren did Paula's depression dramatically lift, allowing her then to enter a state of blessedness. Although she had not been an attentive mother to her own children because of mental and physical illness, she nevertheless received enough benefit from treatment and life experience to become a caring grandmother. Her rhapsodic and protective love affair with her grandchildren became an inspiration to her fellow group members, even those who had no children of their own. In the absence of biological offspring, they were enabled by Paula's example to shower a similar kind of attention on their symbolic children, the products of their callings.

With grandchildren, we get a second chance, free from the pressures of the first time around, to be better parental figures than we were with our own children. Remarkably, our children, when they see us behave more adequately with their children, benefit from this vicarious experience, undoing some of the damage we may have caused them by our earlier deficits. Our children can also teach us to do better by their own examples of parenting. At our best, we are grateful to them for these lessons in child care, which may at first provoke resentment—"Aren't you being too indulgent?"—followed by pride in their competence. Barriers to learning from our children and our patients, not to mention our teachers and therapists, are fundamental barriers to enjoying the blessedness of a spiritual life. The feeling of gratitude to them attests to the expansion of spirit necessary to overcoming these barriers.

Caring Friends

We are blessed when we have a circle of loyal friends who share in our mutual affection. Holding onto some of our friendships from earlier times is a testimony to loyalty and persistence. These personal bonds help us put into perspective early, formative experiences, from times when we were perhaps more fun-seeking but also more imprudent than we have now become. These shared experiences can be, like good early family life, money in the bank; they can serve as part of the endowment whose value, while growing over time, also serves as a baseline to gauge our subsequent development. In addition, gathering around us new friends from our years of maturity affords the richness of an expanding range of connections. To have a network of valued friends is to be blessed exponentially by shared wisdom and trust. Beyond this, their sustained caring protects us from mental and physical illness, as many studies of the preconditions for good health have shown.[95] Lack of a supportive social network is highly associated with vulnerability to illnesses and accidents and poor recovery from them. It is also one of the prime indications for the need to join a therapy group.

The Calling and Character

We are blessed when we have found our calling. To engage in activities that express our most cherished interests and talents and at the same time make a contribution to society is to achieve that blessed state in which we have found work that totally absorbs and fascinates us and enhances our sense of worth. In fact, it is a work from which we derive so much satisfaction that we would do it, if conditions permitted, without monetary compensation or public recognition. Through such work, we transcend the personal ego to answer the call of the higher self within us.

We must not forget that forging a calling also involves strengthening our character. We must resist the temptations to follow a line of work that we do not love or to too readily make compromises in the pursuit of one that we do. Doing so may win us quick approval and yield shortsighted material rewards, but selling out violates the aims of our inmost self and thereby falsifies it. Also, in following the path dictated by our true self, we must not renounce the value of those activities we do easily and naturally and instead believe that only the greatest efforts yield the greatest benefits. In the case of following a calling, the opposite is often true because we are doing what we are ideally suited to do.

Once we affirm the value of exercising our calling, no matter how much it feels like play, we must then assume responsibility for doing it often and well. We must never shrink from our natural tendency to care for the sick, expand the body of knowledge, provide resources for the maimed or indigent, build bridges to connect people and places, invent efficient engines of progress and fuels that spare the environment, compose or play songs of hope and reverence, paint poignant pictures that sensitize us to our fate, or contribute to better methods of education and government—at whatever level of expertise we can render services. Taking on these responsibilities strengthens our character, develops our empathy, and expresses our integrity, the living of which serves as the keystone of the edifice of blessedness.

Integrity, Its Loss, and Its Repair

To have integrity is to be true to one's authentic self and therefore to rarely, and then only strategically and temporarily, violate core values merely for approval or material gain. The wholeness intrinsic to the concept of integrity applies most clearly to human identity and will. Integrity is lost when the will has been broken, leading to the development of a false self. This is most clearly the case when our autonomy has been violated early in life, when we have been forced to knuckle under to harsh demands for obedience and conformity at the expense of exercising our unique, individual interests and talents. We might as children manifest an artistic talent that is derided as a waste of time. Instead we are forced to do busywork, to engage in activities such as sports or heavy manual work for which we have little aptitude, and to renounce any questioning of parental authority, reinforced by the threat of withdrawn love and even physical punishment. For one of my patients, one of the scarce memories of her childhood on a farm was the endless moving of piles of dirt in a wheelbarrow. Poorly coordinated, she was forced to perform this onerous task with threats of physical punishment. A more appropriate contribution to family welfare—she was an excellent knitter and sewer—was never entertained.

Such coercions constitute a form of brainwashing that, in breaking the will, maims the soul by inducing us to forfeit our true self and take on a false one that secures the approval that we cannot live without as dependent children. When we are older and stronger, we can rebuild integrity, repair the broken will, and reclaim our true identity by repeated acts of willful aggression, though always fraught with the apprehension that we will not be able to stand firm if counterattacked. In truth, we may fail many times before we break through and finally throw off the yoke of oppression. It is the goal of the spiritual therapist to provide opportunities for this to happen. One of the essentials is for the therapist to provide not just an auxiliary ego, but an auxiliary will. Later discarding this auxiliary will, after some of its strength and purpose have been incorporated into one's being, is a necessary step in attaining psychological and spiritual maturity.

For example, Richard, whose father was an intimidating, psychotic criminal whom Richard had always feared—with good reason—to confront, spent his days in a state of barely suppressed hostility, never overtly questioning my suggestions and only barely hinting at his reservations. After being repeatedly urged to level with me about his disagreements, he came clean and heatedly told me I was wrong about the reasons he had missed an appointment and that since I had made many mistakes of judgment in the past, he was no longer going to accept my interpretations without carefully examining their rationale. After a sustained rebellion, in reaction to which I held my position without retaliation, Richard settled down and began to take issue with me and other authority figures in a less accusatory manner. After a time, he became a more assertive, self-assured man, more productive and creative than before. A brilliant scientist, he had little use for overtly spiritual talk, but he had little doubt about the excitement he felt in doing his work, which he recognized as a calling that contributed to the social good. In psychodynamic terms, this outcome represented a transference resolution. In spiritual terms, it represented a repair of the will and the rebirth of personal integrity, leading to Richard pursuing his work as a calling. Years after testily throwing off my auxiliary will, he e-mailed me an expression of gratitude for my providing a model of group management that he now drew on in his new expanded role of authority.

A more typical resolution involved Lance, an officer in a venture capital firm. Out of the blue, Lance was informed by his wife Susan that his best friend Kevin had propositioned her; Kevin had declared his longstanding attraction to Susan and claimed that he was prepared to divorce his own wife, Jody, to be with her. Susan declined the invitation and told Lance about it. She didn't know how to handle her future relationship with Kevin and Jody, who had been their best family friends and with whom they had vacationed on several occasions. Lance brought the matter up with his group. Knowing that this betrayal would end his relationship with Kevin and Jody, he felt no need to discuss the matter with either of them. The group pointed out that this passively angry way of handling the issue would leave Susan in an uncomfortable position, but more importantly, it amounted to a missed opportunity to give voice to his true feelings—a goal that had repeatedly come up in connection with how his lack of assertiveness had accounted for the slow progress of his career.

Following a review of the psychodynamics of Lance's difficulty in expressing anger (his father died from a heart attack when he was five, and he short-circuited his grieving by buttoning up all strong feelings and instead becoming the class clown), Lance overcame great apprehension and telephoned Kevin. He told Kevin about his sense of betrayal and the destruction of their friendship; moreover, he stated that Kevin would have to make a full confession to Jody for there ever to be the possibility of reconciliation. Afterward, in a marital session, Susan told Lance how proud she was of him and how protected his action made her feel. Subsequently, Lance began to express himself more directly in every phase of his life. He began to break the habit of always hiding his feelings by making jokes when he was hurt, angry, or merely ambitious. He told the CEO of his company that he expected and deserved to be promoted to a more challenging position. He felt that he had overcome his fear of standing up for his true self and projecting his core values. He had regained the integrity of his will and now was positioned to turn his work into something more expressive of his real values and talents.

Patients as well as therapists typically cannot do this kind of reconstructive work as a solitary undertaking. We all need a guide or mentor reinforced by a caring support system, all of whom believe in our promise and worth as human beings. These helpers help us sort out our authentic interests and values and give support for taking the requisite actions to repair the assertive will, strengthen character, and thereby move toward spiritual health.

Having integrity is further defined by the expression of our authenticity and the moral values intrinsic to it. The result is a true self as opposed to a false self acting in bad faith. The moral face of integrity is being truthful, honest, and steadfast in our values and loyalties and always treating others, in Kant's phrase, as ends in themselves. That is, we must treat them as intrinsically valuable beings, who are not to be manipulated or exploited for our gain at their expense—in short, they are not to be used. Achieving the integrity of an authentic identity requires first that we reconcile or integrate conflicting aspects of our personality so that we can present a united, effective, truthful self to others, free of artifice and intent to mislead.

Only for dire and temporarily strategic reasons are we allowed to violate any of the following principles: We must not deny our ethnic and racial origins by playing a false part tricked out with fake accent and bearing, nor may we pretend to political and philosophical positions that do not reflect our true feelings. We cannot simulate a form of masculinity or femininity, a gender identity that we do not legitimately own. *Whatever* we are, we must, in the interests of authenticity, come out as *who* we really are. This goal of a spiritual therapy can be formulated in this affirmation of self: *I shall become who I really am.*[96] These words can form the basis of a meditation or chant that focuses the will, in the effort to achieve blessedness, to become an authentic self and to express its true purpose in a calling.

Integrating Conflicting Parts of the Personality

The task of reconciling conflicting aspects of the personality is, quite obviously, less strenuous if we come from the mainstream of a homogeneous society whose values, religion, and ethnicity are commonly shared. Even in this case, however, unusual talents and interests may become manifest and set us apart. Overt expression of these differences, in violation of social conformity, calls for a degree of courage that is essential to integrity and authenticity. In multiethnic societies such as North America and parts of Europe, the labor of integration among the multiplicity of racial and cultural groups is a much more demanding task.

For example, who am I? I am all of the following: a rural Southerner by birth and early development; a transplanted East Coast urban American; a firmly identified, partially observant Jew, less out of an exclusive theological commitment than in honor of a rich cultural heritage; a retired but once on-call physician who could be reached at almost any hour; a broad-gauged, multidisciplinary psychiatrist who would use any approach that had been shown to work; a social liberal supportive of a large safety net ultimately providing health care, education, and material security to all those in need; an economic conservative who abhors waste and feather-bedding; a heterosexual in touch with his feminine self; a believer in market capitalism with curbs on grave inequities; a supporter of public ownership or subsidization of utilities, transportation systems, and the arts; an intellectual about comparative belief systems, meaning that arguments for their validity should be subjected to rigorous examination of their basis in faith or reason; a pragmatist about survival techniques, especially in reference to new techniques for disease prevention and cure; an intuitionist about moral-spiritual values, in full recognition that these intuitions must be subjected to critical thought because they sometimes turn out to be illusory distortions; a believer in a higher organizing energy or intelligence called Spirit, cognizant that such a belief may well be encoded in our brains through the evolutionary process; and an agnostic about a personal God who directly speaks to us and answers our prayers. To be authentic, people like me, the products of diverse backgrounds, beliefs, and cultures, have to come up with a workable resolution of all these competing claims on our true identity. We have to start by admitting that we have such conflicting attributes. Then the sifting and winnowing, the prioritizing, must be undertaken. And we do not apologize for changing any of these defining beliefs or biases, not for self-aggrandizement, but to take account of new learning.

For instance, although I do not deny the importance of any of the aforementioned facets of my personality, some of them are more essential to my identity than others, manifesting themselves more forcefully and with greater consistency. Therefore, to achieve authenticity, I try not to pander by, at different times, claiming one attribute and denying others to win approval. I try not to create doubt as to where I basically stand and what I stand for. First and foremost, I am a human being who tries to behave honestly and considerately but who does not always succeed, even though I continue to work at it. I am an American who believes in the fundamental values of this democratic society, despite all its faults and its capacity to go astray in social programming and waging war. Yet I believe that the collective "we" will ultimately use the political system to right the listing ship of state. My identity is as a physician first and psychiatrist second. With my extensive medical education, I always strive to be attentive to the health of the whole person and to new developments in the treatment of both mind and body. As a social progressive and economic conservative, I think both agendas must be rationally curbed to minimize social inequities and economic waste. Because we are living in a dangerous world, I believe in strong agencies of defense. All in all, I come out as a political progressive who believes in the equal spiritual worth of every member of society and who hopes we are ready to elect talented leaders from heretofore minority groups, such as women, gays, African Americans, Hispanics, and Jews, whose minority status might make them more sensitive and empathetic than mainstream citizens to the needs and perceptions of different nationalities with whom we interact. If only I could remain true to these principles more fully and more of the time, I would feel more worthy of the sense of blessedness that I currently enjoy and hope to augment.

Most of the time, I sense there is an intelligent principle, force, or energy, which I call Spirit, that permeates and sustains the physical world and shapes the course of human history. Yet its force of destiny leaves room for each of us to develop a measure of free will, thereby making it virtually impossible to accurately predict the details of historical change and evolution. Also, to the extent that we can act freely, limitations on which have been previously discussed, we become morally responsible for our actions and thereby are held accountable and deserving of rewards and punishment. I believe that the main events of creation and destruction, particularly the world's beginnings and evolution, are not just chance events; rather, they are often permeated with a purpose that I do not fully grasp. I think that our individual minds are playing a part in the Spirit's becoming aware of its own unfolding, so that it may guide its own future evolution to ever higher spiritual and material peaks. I follow Teilhard de Chardin in his way of thinking about evolution as progressing toward a spiritual unity.[97] At the same time, I recognize that the integrity of modern science requires that we eliminate such considerations from the teaching and pursuit of scientific knowledge, at least as currently defined. (Thanks for sharing, Gene).

The Cynicism of an Indifferent World

Because it is largely constituted of the highest common denominator of all human minds, Spirit, as I see it, is neither hostile nor indifferent to the human enterprise. Should we attribute to Spirit such indifference or hostility, we cannot help but succumb to a form of skepticism or cynicism that cuts us off from having a spiritual life and its sense of blessedness. In fact, living in a world of chance instead of enchantment is the very opposite of feeling spiritually blessed. To feel blessed with its accompanying joy and peace of mind, we must believe that the organizing force of the universe is, in fact, a benign, progressive force whose direction we can align ourselves with, either by spontaneous heightening of consciousness or by meditation, prayer, visualization, and other spiritual practices. At such times of heightened awareness, we cannot help but belong to the community of the faithful, even though we may be reluctant to use the word God to refer to the object of faith because we have doubts as to its personal nature. In any case, spiritual believers that I identify with do not think it appropriate to speak of a divinity, certainly with a name bearing such connotations as 'God' outside places of worship. We do not believe that religious faith of any denomination should be promoted in public schools, courts, or the political marketplace.

Absolute Values

In stressing the unique values of each individual's true self, I do not wish to be misunderstood as making the case for moral relativism. Quite to the contrary, I believe that all individuals whose connection to Spirit has not been obliterated by past traumas or genetic miscarriages share a common self at their core being and therefore a common set of absolute values. Some of these are the "shall not" values having to do with killing, harming, deceiving, stealing, and coercing without overriding cause. Others are the "shall do" values having to do with developing potentials, treating others as ourselves, taking actions to repair the world, and expressing gratitude for what we have been given. Beyond these absolutes and others unmentioned, there are relative values about which reasonable people can disagree, such as whether to vote for the left or the right, to support egalitarianism or elitism, to be pro-choice or pro-life, to engage in preemptive or only defensive wars. The seeming moral relativism of having tolerance for others who hold beliefs that we "know" to be mistaken but know we cannot disprove is, paradoxically, an absolute value.

Part of our blessedness is to live in a beautiful world with its great variety of flowers, streams, waterfalls, and mountains; to have pets who love us as we love them; and to live near forests full of wondrous plants, trees, and wild animals. Therefore, it is an absolute value that we do everything in our power to conserve and develop these environments and their life forms. Whether we belong to the organizations of the environmental movement or simply do our private part to preserve the world and its many species of plants and animals, we must recognize that our fate is inextricably bound up with the prospering of the planet, no less a manifestation of Spirit than our own existence. We must do what we can to reduce the destructive by-products of manufacturing and economic operations that lead to dangerous pollutions of the environment and unequal distributions of wealth in the absence of creating real products of worth to the living world.

We must become aware that every walk or ride we set out on can and should become a treasurable experience of the multiplicity of nature's bounty. In some ways, these natural monuments far exceed the beauty of any museum collection of human artifacts. And yet we can also experience the expressive power of these artifacts, which, at their best, tap into the universal truth and power behind all forms of creation. There are films, symphonies, songs, statues, gardens, and buildings that reach the exalted level of spiritual inspiration. Thankfully, they occupy spaces in cities, museums, and parks, installations that we can enjoy and be enriched by, thus contributing to our sense of blessedness.

Joyful Summation

To conclude that the world, however beautiful or pleasure-giving, is indifferent or even hostile to our well-being is clearly the opposite of feeling blessed. It is tantamount to being disillusioned and nihilistic about the purpose and meaning of life. The answer we give to this central question—is the world here for human perception, enjoyment, and betterment (a positive answer is the so-called anthropic principle[98]), or is it the product of blind material forces that have no reference to human aspirations?—defines whether or not we are consciously spiritual. The spiritual answer commits us to feeling gratitude for being put on this earth and given the gifts that our mere conscious existence provides.

We are blessed when we can ungrudgingly give gratitude to all who have improved our lives. We feel grateful to the inventors, scientists, thinkers, and spiritual and political leaders who have inspired humankind to lead a better, more fulfilling life; grateful to the mentors who have shown us the path and guided us along it to fulfill our potential; grateful to the great artists who have filled our world with works of beauty and meaning; and grateful to friends for loving and inspiring us and to our parents for bringing us into the world and tending to our infantile needs, no matter how far short they have fallen in their care, providing, of course, that they have tried their best and not intentionally and gravely abused us.

We are blessed to live in a country that gives men and women the freedom to believe or not believe in a higher power, that has a relatively impartial rule of law, that has the potential to afford freedom of opportunity to all who come to its shores, and that integrates successive waves of immigrants into the fabric of society. Despite the fact that the disabled and underprivileged are sometimes consigned to live in dismal ghettos of neglect, the spirit of the nation is poised to recognize when the social safety net has been torn and to swing the pendulum toward effecting repairs. We are privileged to live in a society that has the capacity to self-correct such lapses in achieving its ideals.

I feel personally blessed to have practiced a healing calling and to have been free to do it in a personal, idiosyncratic rather than officially prescribed way. I feel blessed that early in life I experienced the tugs of the moral law within that helped me battle inborn racial prejudices and allowed me to appreciate the great achievements of our finest human exemplars. I am grateful for the heightened experiences of great music and art that I can share with my friends, family, and patients. And I feel endless gratitude for being able to experience the beauties of the natural world and to understand the sciences that help us make sense of some of its workings.

To whom or what are we to be grateful for all these blessings? Is there, as I believe, a creative, healing will behind this blessed world, which calls for our deepest appreciation? Or as a spate of books have recently argued,[99] are we just terribly lucky winners of a chance lottery in the cosmos? The precise nature of this good fortune is beyond our capacity to describe and understand. But I intuitively sense that there is a spiritual force that lies behind and animates the living world and gives it purpose and meaning. How else do we explain "the moral law within and the starry skies above?" Is this belief only a myth or an illusion deriving from the sense of an aggregate world mind, the integration of all minds? If it is, then we must be grateful for the imaginative capacity to create such a myth and to sustain such an illusion. And those of us who share in this illusion should feel blessed to be able to fend off disillusionment and despair when we face the inevitable losses of this short biological life.

We may call this spiritual agency whatever we like—the collective unconscious, fate, Eros, evolution, inborn genetic structure, God, the Holy Spirit—but whatever we call it, my hope is that we will invest it with purpose so that we feel gratitude for its operation in the world. In the absence of gratitude, there is no sense of blessedness. We do not wish on anyone the tunnel vision that leads to disenchantment with the mysterious unfolding of the life of sentient beings and their cosmos.

But of course death and loss dig the hole of despair we must all climb out of to reach the state of blessedness, for we will not have traveled far along the pathway of our lives before we fall into the potholes of failures and losses, whose pain may at times overwhelm our sense of joy. And despite all efforts to deny it, we cannot fail to realize that ultimately we will die. (Kafka even said that the meaning of life is that it will end!!) Despite this tragic sense of the cycles of life and death, we must assert our will, firm up our resolve, and set off again on our spiritual path as it stretches out to the horizon.

It is the job of our living spirit to honor our mothers and fathers for giving us the gift of life, to own our true self, to merge it with the higher Self, and then to obey its promptings to gratefully give back to the world for everything we have been given and if at all possible to appreciate that the gifts far exceed the deprivations and abuses that we inevitably suffer. These are the ultimate requirements of leading a spiritual life and entering the state of blessedness.

ENDNOTES

Introduction

1. See Immanuel Kant, *Critique of Pure Reason*, translated by Norman Kemp Smith (Macmillan, 1929); *Critique of Practical Reason*, ed. Lewis W. Beck (University of Chicago, 1949); John Rawls, *A Theory of Justice* (Belknap, 1971); Derek Parfit, *On What Matters*, Vol. 1 (Oxford, 2011).

2. Abraham Maslow, *Toward a Psychology of Being*, 2nd ed. (Van Nostrand, 1968).

3. Jay Haley gives a scintillating account of Erickson's methods from the point of view of Palo Alto communications theory and his own directive, strategic family therapy. See Haley's *Uncommon Therapy: The Psychiatric Techniques of Milton H. Erickson, M.D.* (Norton, 1993).

4. Although it has some ideas in common, my outlook in this book tries to be more comprehensive than the optimistic school of "positive psychology," developed by Martin Seligman and his followers. Jonathan Haidt's *The Happiness Hypothesis* (Basic Books, 2006) and *The Righteous Mind* (Pantheon, 2012) are excellent accounts of some of the fruits of this approach as applied to defining the prerequisites for achieving happiness and a life of moral worth. I particularly appreciate Haidt's efforts to empirically validate the prerequisites for happiness in research studies in the first book and his thoughts about the basis for moral and political harmony in the second.

5. Freud proposed in his 1930 monograph, *Civilization and Its Discontents*, The Standard Edition of the Complete Psychological works of Sigmund Freud (vol.21, Hogarth, 1961) that the civilizing trends of modern society serve to repress the instinctual life and therefore lead to the "discontents" of neurotic suffering, a restrictive idea rejected by the expansive, spiritual thrust of my work. Yet Freud was certainly right

that without a spiritual life that transcends instinctual and materialistic needs, the constraints imposed by civilization cannot be easily, much less expansively, overcome.

Chapter 1

6. Steven Levenkron, *Treating and Overcoming Anorexia Nervosa*, Warner, 1982. This is Levenkron's standard account of his approach. But if memory serves me, the patient presented me with his novelized account, *The Best Little Girl in the World*, 1979. The author might not approve of my interpretation of his work, but the uses I put it to were inevitably filtered through my own work on setting limits. See G.M. Abroms, *Setting Limits,* Archives of General Psychiatry, **19**:113-119, 1968.

7. For an interesting account of this tactic, a must for any therapist or parent with an out-of-control offspring, see Sandor Ferenczi, "On Taming a Wild Horse," in *Final Contributions to the Problems and Methods of Psycho-analysis* (Hogarth Press, 1955).

8. "Serendip" is an old name for Ceylon, now Sri Lanka, whose accidental discovery is recounted in *The Three Princes of Serendip*.

9. Carl Jung, *Synchronicity: An Acausal Connecting Principle* (Princeton, 1973).

10. Paul Kammerer's laws of coincidences are discussed extensively in Arthur Koestler's popularization *The Roots of Coincidence* (Random House, 1972).

11. Jill Bolte Taylor, *My Stroke of Insight* (Viking, 2008), p. 69.

12. F. M. Cornford (trans.), *The Republic of Plato* (Oxford, 1945), p. 227.

13. Henri Bergson, *Creative Evolution* (Random House, 1944).

14. Pierre Teilhard de Chardin, *The Phenomenon of Man* (Harper, 1975).

15. Cognitive-behavioral therapy was pioneered by Aaron T. Beck at the University of Pennsylvania. His work in treating depression is summarized in Beck et al., *Cognitive Therapy of Depression* (Guilford, 1979). A comprehensive account of its modern formulation can be found in S. G. Hofmann, *An Introduction to Modern CBT* (Wiley-Blackwell, 2011).

Chapter 2

16. See A. Horowitz and J. Wakefield, *The Loss of Sadness: How Psychiatry Transformed Normal Sadness into Depressive Disorder* (Oxford, 2007).

17. Many have questioned this "rush to happiness" as a very shallow, unnatural quest. See Eric Wilson, *Against Happiness* (Farrar, Strauss, and Giroux, 2008).

18. The idea of a paradigm shift was introduced by T. S. Kuhn in his landmark work, *The Structure of Scientific Revolutions* (U. of Chicago, 1962). He traced how in hard science, a whole set of events may lead to a radical change in the basic assumptions about the nature of scientific truth. This revolutionary change in framework occurred when Newton's assumption of absolute space and time gave way to Einstein's theory of relativity. I think psychotherapy has undergone a paradigm shift in the past half century as the psychogenic paradigm has given way to a multicausal biopsychosocial paradigm. In one sense, I am recommending a new paradigm that also takes account of spiritual influences.

19. Jerome Frank, in *Persuasion and Healing,* (Johns Hopkins, 1962), was one of the first psychiatrists to stress the importance of persuasion in all forms of attitude and behavior change, applying not only to psychotherapy but also to indoctrination and religious conversion. He also recognized these processes inevitably fostered value-changes in the targeted populations.

20. Primal screaming and "body work" are typical of faddist treatments without objective evidence of accrued benefits. In fact, they sometimes lead to psychiatric casualties requiring crisis intervention.

21. This verdict was delivered by Nietzsche in his monograph *The Gay Science*, perhaps better translated now as *The Joyful Science*, in which he proposes his alternative to traditional religious belief. See any of Walter Kaufmann's books on the philosopher, such as the *Portable Nietzsche* (Viking, 1954).

22. The most succinct statement of this characteristic form of mid-twentieth-century scientific empiricism can be found in A. J. Ayer's *Language, Truth, and Logic* (Dover, 1946).

23. See Wendy Mogel's *The Blessings of a Skinned Knee* (Penguin, 2001) for a summary of these values as applied to child rearing and family values.

24. Erich Fromm's *Escape from Freedom* (Farrar and Rinehart, 1941) makes the case that human beings have a propensity to give up their free will to avoid the guilt and shame that its exercise inevitably gives rise to. This escape from freedom results in the formation of a false, hollow self that is socially conformist and submissive to even the most irrational, abusive forms of authority, as happened in Nazi Germany but as is all too frequently manifested in our own political process and in the formation of cults as well.

Chapter 3

25. In one of its many formulations, Kant's categorical imperative enjoins us to treat others as ends in themselves, not as means to our or others' interests.

26. See Benjamin Wolberg, *The Technique of Psychotherapy*, 2nd ed. (Grune and Stratton, 1967). The discussion of short-term therapy in part 2, pp. 916-930, is particularly illuminating.

27. American Psychiatric Association, *Diagnostic and Statistical Manual of Mental Disorders*, 5th ed. (APA, 2013).

28. I am referring to Don D. Jackson, MD (1922-1968), winner of many awards, founder and first director of the Mental Research Institute in Palo Alto, California, and major contributor to the family therapy

movement. He is credited with formulating the concepts of "family homeostasis" and the "double bind" theory of schizophrenia. He apparently took his own life at the apogee of his professional success only hours after his forty-sixth birthday.

29. This quote comes from Walter Isaacson's masterful biography, *Einstein: His Life and Universe* (Simon and Schuster, 2007), p. 388. It is contained in Einstein's letter to a sixth grader, found in the chapter titled "Einstein's God." His God, as indicated in the quote, is by no means the personal God of organized religion; rather, it is an impersonal organizing spiritual force, whose first conception is attributed to Spinoza. For such radical ideas, this founding philosopher of the Enlightenment was excommunicated by his Amsterdam synagogue in 1655, at age twenty-three, and his books were later put on the Catholic Church's *Index of Forbidden Books*.

30. See Rupert Sheldrake, *The Presence of the Past: Morphic Resonance and the Habits of Nature* (Vintage, 1989).

31. See Victor Frankl, *Man's Search for Meaning* (Pocket Books, 1984).

32. Otto Rank, *Will Therapy and Truth and Reality* (Knopf, 1972).

33. This refers to the remarkable story of the fraudulent memoir of one "Binyamin Wilkomirski," whose lectures and writings were even sponsored by the US Holocaust Museum before his true origins and counterfeit account were demythologized. See Mark Weber's piece in the *Journal of Historical Review* **17** (1998).

34. Erik H. Erikson, *Childhood and Society*, 2nd ed. (Norton, 1963).

35. Heinz Kohut, *The Analysis of the Self* (International Universities Press, 1971).

36. Immanuel Kant, *The Critique of Pure Reason* (Macmillan, 1959). This is Kant's concept of the *ding-an-sich*—that is, ultimate reality that has not been transformed by the limitations of our sense organs and brain structure. Therefore, it cannot be an object of empirical knowledge; it

can only be intuited. According to Schopenhauer, this ultimate reality is Will, the attributes of which are attainable by introspection rather than external perception. Unfortunately, this thrilling and profound insight did not save Schopenhauer from a pervasive pessimism about the human condition.

Chapter 4

37. An important exception was the eminent psychologist Rollo May, whose *Love and Will* (Norton, 1969) argued eloquently for the will's importance in realizing the human potential for love and fulfillment.

38. See Ernest Nagel and James Newman, *Gödel's Proof* (New York University Press, 1973), for an explanation of the proof that not all the true statements about a subject, such as the earth's present climate, can be deduced from a coherent set of initial conditions, no matter how extensive the set. The implication is that other factors, such as unforeseen human choices leading, for example, to global climate change, may throw off the predictions. Among the unforeseen factors, this time a mitigating factor, might be a social fit of conscience, a spiritual phenomenon, that leads to widespread human restriction on carbon dioxide and methane emissions. The unpredictability of empirical phenomena is further amplified by the confounding observer effects addressed by Heisenberg's uncertainty principle and the general probabilistic nature of quantum physics, as mentioned earlier.

39. I have discussed the general topic of freedom versus determinism in an earlier work, *The Freedom of the Self* (Plenum, 1993).

40. *Webster's Third New International Dictionary* (Merriam-Webster, 1963).

41. Walter Isaacson's *Einstein: His Life and Universe* (Simon and Schuster, 2007) gives an exceptionally clear popular account of Einstein's religious beliefs. As mentioned earlier, his was an aloof, Spinozan deity who set the world in motion but did not intervene day-to-day. An interesting question, posed by my friend Richard Wernick, is whether or not the expanding matter of the Big Bang was already imbued with some form of intelligent organization.

42. See Rupert Sheldrake, *The Presence of the Past: Morphic Resonance and the Habits of Nature* (Vintage, 1988). Sheldrake, an English biologist, floats the idea that memories are stored not only within brains but also between brains in morphic fields or memory nets. This is an interesting model for the possibility of nongenetic racial and tribal transmission patterns that reside in what Jung termed the collective unconscious.

43. J. W. N. Sullivan, *Beethoven: His Spiritual Development* (Mentor Books, 1949. first published 1927). In accounting for the growing communicative power and complexity of Beethoven's music going from his early to middle to late periods, Sullivan defined "spiritual" in terms of an enhanced neural integrative power. As a scientist and mathematician, he clearly found it difficult to escape the box of scientific materialism. Nevertheless, this book had a powerful influence on twentieth-century music lovers who were trying to ascribe an extra-musical significance to great pieces of music.

44. "SSRIs" stands for selective serotonin reuptake inhibitors, such as Prozac, Zoloft, Celexa, and Lexapro. "SNRIs" stands for selective norepinephrine reuptake inhibitors, such as Effexor and Pristiq. The latter, which also contain an SSRI component, tend to give patients greater energy.

45. See Herbert Benson, *The Relaxation Response* (Harper Collins, 2000), a popularization of Transcendental Meditation as applied to treating hypertension and heart disease. Also see Lawrence LeShan, *How to Meditate* (Little Brown, 1974).

46. I am indebted to my colleague Carl Whitaker, now deceased, for this image of the roots, trunk, and limbs of a multicausal mental realm.

Chapter 5

47. I am referring here to the effects of low-dose antipsychotic medication on cognitive focusing in nonpsychotic as well as psychotic individuals.

48. Joe McGinniss's *Fatal Vision* (Signet, 1983) is the trailblazing account of the "true crime" genre. McGinniss was concerned only with establishing

McDonald's innocence or guilt and therefore did not go beyond the question of whether he was telling the truth or lying.

49. Eugene Abroms, *The Freedom of the Self* (Plenum, 1993).

50. See Flora Schreiber, *Sybil* (Penguin, 1973); Corbett Thigpen and Hervey Cleckley, *The Three Faces of Eve* (Popular Library, 1957).

51. Schopenhauer, *The World as Will and Representation*, 2 vols., trans. Payne (Dover, 1969).

52. Abroms, *The Freedom of the Self*, op.cit.

53. Gene M. Abroms, "Setting Limits," *Archives of General Psychiatry* 19 (1968):113-119.

54. Carl Rogers, founder of the school of nondirective therapy, claimed that the therapist's essential tasks were limited to providing clarifying, reflective feedback and "unconditional positive regard" and did not include providing restraints and limits. Rogers apparently had never treated a ragingly suicidal or homicidal patient. Following is the classic Rogerian spoof: Client says, "I'm going to kill myself." Therapist says, "So you are feeling self-destructive." Client jumps out ten-story window. Therapist reflectively comments, "Plop!" Or there is the following. Question: "Why are you letting that stranger sitting next to you fondle your breasts?" Answer: "That's his problem."

Chapter 6

55. The American Psychiatric Association's *Diagnostic and Statistical Manual*, 5th edition, 2013. This is the reference manual for the clinical criteria of the standard psychiatric disorders.

56. Gustave Le Bon, *The Crowd*, 2nd ed. (Cherokee Publishing, 1982).

57. Sigmund Freud, *Group Psychology and the Analysis of the Ego*, Complete Psychological Works of Sigmund Freud, Standard Edition, vol. 18 (1955).

58. Freud, *Civilization and Its Discontents*, Standard Edition, vol. 21 (1961).

59. Gene M Abroms, "Defining Milieu Therapy," *Archives of General Psychiatry* 21 (1969); GM Abroms and NS Greenfield, eds., *The New Hospital Psychiatry* (Academic Press, 1971).

60. For a discussion of the holy or numinous qualities of spiritual experience, there is no better source than Rudolf Otto's *The Idea of the Holy*, 2nd ed. (Oxford, 1958).

Chapter 7

61. The USA Patriot Act, signed by President George W. Bush in October 2001 in the wake of the September 11 terrorist attack on the United States and extended by President Obama in May 2011, authorizes the gathering of intelligence by conducting wiretaps, examining financial records, and holding or deporting suspected terrorists, foreign or domestic, without customary due process.

62. The Durham Rule of 1954 was authored by Judge David Bazelon, a strong advocate for the rights of the mentally ill. He was the senior member of the DC Court of Appeals in the case of *Durham v. United States*.

63. Immanuel Kant, "Foundations of the Metaphysics of Morals," in *Critique of Practical Reason*, ed. Lewis Beck (University of Chicago, 1949).

64. Sam Harris, *Free Will* (Free Press, 2012).

65. Hannah Arendt, *Eichmann in Jerusalem: A Report on the Banality of Evil* (Penguin, 1963).

66. See Daniel Kahneman, *Thinking, Fast and Slow*, Farrar, Strauss, and Giroux, (2011); and Malcolm Gladwell, *Blink*, Little, Brown (2005). Neither author is primarily interested in moral judgment as the product of fast, intuitive thinking. But both emphasize the importance of snap

judgments. Kahneman concentrates on the distortions fast thinking yields without the balancing affects of slow, critical thinking. Gladwell emphasizes that snap judgments often prove more reliable than careful weighing of evidence. He refrains from calling them intuitions. I imagine this is because he wants to lay claim to their empirically objective nature.

67. See Gary Becker, *Human Capital,* 3rd edition (U of Chicago, 1993).

68. Chuck Klosterman, "The Ethicist," *New York Times Magazine*, July 22, 2012, p. 20

69. G. M. Abroms, "Setting Limits," *Archives of General Psychiatry* 19 (1968): 113-119.

70. This is quite obviously a personal judgment, but I think it is no accident that with few exceptions the most acclaimed twentieth-century composers and artists either were refugees from Nazi Germany-Austria or were native Americans, Brits, or Russians.

71. *The Autobiography of Mark Twain*, vol. 1 (U of California, 2010).

72. Saul Bellow, *Mr. Sammler's Planet* (Viking Press, 1970), p. 313.

73. Edward O. Wilson, the eminent pioneer of sociobiology, makes the best possible case for the origins of the moral sense in the facts of evolutionary biology. See his *Consilience: The Unity of Knowledge* (Knopf, 1998) for a readable account of his position. Note that he slips in many undefined spiritual terms in making his argument, which testifies as much to his tacit spirituality as to the validity of his argument.

74. The history of the philosophy known as idealism, which maintains that the physical world is fundamentally the mind-stuff of ideas and sense-data rather than the matter-stuff of objects, goes back to the pre-Socratic philosophers. George Berkeley (1685-1753), an Irish philosopher, is perhaps the best-known post-Renaissance proponent of this viewpoint, although the interpretation of his viewpoint as casting

doubt on whether the tree falls in the forest if no one happens to be observing the event is simplistic and an invitation to parody. Modern quantum physics places the idea on firmer ground, so to speak.

75. Phil Jackson, *The Last Season: A Team in Search of Its Soul* (Penguin, 2004).

76. Wilhelm Reich, *Character Analysis* (FSG, 1961, originally published in German, 1933). His theory of "orgone energy accumulators," or what came to be known as orgone boxes, was described in many left-wing journals of the day, such as *The New Republic*, and was subjected to attempts at empirical validation by no less a figure than Albert Einstein, with results that were quite disappointing to its proponents.

77. *Webster's Third New International Dictionary* (Merriam-Webster, 1966).

Chapter 8

78. *Webster's Third New International Dictionary* (Merriam-Webster, 1966).

79. Roberto Assagioli, *Psychosynthesis* (Viking Press, 1965).

Chapter 9

80. See *Baghwan Shree Rajneesh: The True Sage* (Rajneesh Foundation, 1976) for a characteristic work.

81. Swami Prabhavanda and Christopher Isherwood, trans., *Bhagavad-Gita* (New American Library, 1954).

82. See the work of J. B. Rhine, for example *Extra Sensory Perception* (Branden, 1973), and the publications of the Rhine Research Center. Rupert Sheldrake is perhaps the best-known contemporary proponent of parapsychological phenomena; see *The Presence of the Past: Morphic Resonance and the Habits of Nature* (Vintage, 1988).

83. Daniel Kahneman *Thinking, Fast and Slow,*(op.cit); Malcolm Gladwell, *Blink* (op.cit).

84. As previously discussed, this phenomenon is named after William of Occam, a medieval English philosopher who said, "It is vain to do with more what can be done with fewer." As Bertrand Russell put it in his *A History of Western Philosophy* (Simon and Schuster, 1945), "if everything in some science can be interpreted without assuming this or that hypothetical entity, there is no ground for assuming it." As must be obvious, I believe this is destructively reductionist thinking.

85. Erich Fromm, *Escape from Freedom*, op. cit.

86. Heinz Kohut, *The Analysis of the Self* (International Universities Press, 1971).

Chapter 10

87. W. G. Plaut, ed., *The Torah: A Modern Commentary* (UAHC, 1981), pp. 20-23.

88. Malcolm Gladwell, *Outliers* (Little, Brown, 2008). The author argues that success depends not only on being born into the right circumstances in terms of human capital but also on putting in at least 10,000 hours in practicing a craft or work.

89. As already mentioned, this is another useful concept from Gladwell's book *Blink*, which refers to intuitive snap judgments whose validity is hard to account for by empirical observation alone.

90. Bruno Bettelheim ran a seemingly successful psychoanalytically based school for adolescents in Chicago during the post—World War II years. Subsequently, students came forward to accuse him of abusive, corporeal punishment. His prized credentials, including Viennese training in psychoanalysis from Freud's disciples, also turned out to be less than solidly based. It is shocking to remember how revered he was in therapy circles when one considers his life may have been based on a false self. Nevertheless, to complicate the issue, his book interpreting the meaning of fairy tales, *The Uses of Enchantment* (Random House, 1976), is nothing less than enchanting itself, although Bettelheim was accused of plagiarism in writing it. In the mind, creativity occupies a place right

next to criminality and psychosis.

91. Gurdjieff was a Sufi-trained Tartar who was alleged to have "mind control" over his acolytes in various ventures, including dance groups and communal living experiments. Apparently, judging from the casualty rate, this mind control of others did not involve his own self-control. For a flavor of the man and his journeying, see his illuminating work *Meetings with Remarkable Men* (Dutton, 1969).

Chapter 11

92. The importance of our relationship to death is a central tenet of Tibetan Buddhism, as brilliantly discussed by Sogyal Rinpoche in *The Tibetan Book of Living and Dying* (HarperCollins, 1994).

93. Linda Noble Topf, *You Are Not Your Illness* (Fireside Books, 1995).

94. George Herbert Mead, *Mind, Self, and Society* (University of Chicago, 1934).

95. T. R. Holmes and R. H. Rahe have done the major work on the stressors leading to illness and the value of social support in warding off the consequences of stress. The Holmes and Rahe Stress Scale is described in their landmark work: Holmes and Rahe, "The Social Readjustment Rating Scale," *Journal of Psychosomatic Research* 11, no. 2 (1967): 213-218.

96. This formula for a meditation practice derives from the biblical passage in which God affirms, "I am that which I am." Arthur Green in his *Ehyeh: A Kabbalah for Tomorrow* (2004) translates the Hebrew word Ehyeh as "I will be," which fits better with the notion that our higher or true Self is always in the process of becoming.

97. Pierre Teilhard de Chardin, *The Phenomenon of Man* (Harper and Row, 1959).

98. J. D. Barrow and F. J. Tipler, *The Anthropic Cosmological Principle* (Oxford, 1986).

99. See Richard Dawkins, *The God Delusion*, Bantam, 2006; Christopher Hitchens, *God Is Not Great*, Twelve Books, 2007; and Sam Harris, *Letter to a Christian Nation* (Vintage 2007). What these books have in common is rejection of a conception of a higher power sufficiently anthropomorphic and concrete as to be irrelevant to the thinking of most thoughtful, modern believers in a spiritual reality.

INDEX

A

Abbott, Jack, 136–137
Abilify (antipsychotic), 76
absolute values, 179, 241–242
absolution, 96, 109, 151, 154
abulia, 72, 78
abusers, steps to overcome workings of, 95–97
acausal connecting principle, 6
acting-out
    identification of pattern of, 95–96, 98
    stopping of, 96, 98
acupuncture, 201
addictive disorders/personalities, 77, 110, 126, 130, 230
adoption, 232
advocacy, 146
affects, loss of control of, 184–185
Al (case example), 101–102, 107, 108
Albert (case example), 174–175
Alcoholics Anonymous (AA), 7, 77, 149, 187. *See also* twelve-step programs
Alexander, Mr. (case example), 26–27
"Allegory of the Cave" (Plato), 8, 198
alter egos, 84, 92
altruism, 10, 48, 93
amends
    making of, 149, 150
    possibility of lesser amends, 152–153

treatment when amends cannot be made, 151–152
Amin, Idi, 162
anger-management techniques, 188
anthropic principle, 242
anti-cultural bias, as unacceptable in spiritual healer, 129
antidepressants, 20, 22, 25, 26, 76, 105, 115
anti-instincts, 67
anti-intellectual bias, as unacceptable in spiritual healer, 129
antipsychotics, 76, 86, 99, 105, 131
anti-religious bias, as unacceptable in spiritual healer, 128–129
antisocial personalities, 39, 126, 130–131, 140, 161, 230
anti-spiritual pathology, 130–131
anxiolytics, 105
appetites, loss of control of, 180–182
Arendt, Hannah, 139
arrogance, 168, 180, 184
artistic ramifications (of spiritual therapy), 17
artistic-spiritual realm, 24
artists
    sources of best works of, 57
    unconscious sources of works of, 49
arts, 209
Assagioli, Roberto, 187
assertiveness, work therapy and, 120–121
assertiveness training, 121

athletic teams, as characterized by spiritual caring, 230
attention, focusing of, 199–200
authenticity, 17, 56, 170, 171, 237, 238, 239
auxiliary ego, 236
auxiliary will, 236

B

B, Mr. (case example), 185
Bach, Johann Sebastian, 37, 126, 147
basketball, changes in, 23
Beck, Aaron T., 165
Beethoven, Ludwig van, 20, 37, 72, 147, 195
behavioral hologram, 107, 108
being, ground of, 48, 57
being needs, x
belief(s)
    Eastern belief systems/wisdom, 196, 230
    in God, 10, 28, 199, 241
    making transition to positive beliefs, 10
    rational belief system, 163
    as spiritual term, 51
    tolerance vs. dogmatic belief, 137
Bellow, Saul, 148
belonging, 40, 66, 78, 79–80, 227, 232
Ben (case example), 218
Bennett, John G., Jr., 89
Bergson, Henri, 11, 127
Bernard (case example), 158–160, 161
Bettelheim, Bruno, 222
better angels, as other name for Spirit, 58
Bhagavad-Gita, 191
biological drives, 63

biological mortality, 227
blessedness
    absolute values, 241–242
    calling and character, 234
    caring friends, 234
    cynicism of an indifferent world, 240–241
    family belonging, adoption, and special importance of grandchildren, 232
    integrating conflicting parts of personality, 238–240
    integrity, its loss, its repair, 235–238
    joyful summation, 242–244
    love and creation/destruction of spirit, 231
    love partners, 229
    overview, 227–228
    platonic spiritual love, 229–231
The Blessings of a Skinner Knee (Mogel), 30
blind spots (of patient), 98, 101
blinks, 139, 193, 218
blocked will, 59, 75, 76, 80, 83
Blue Cross, 123
borderline personalities, 104, 113, 114, 126, 154, 197
bound will, 72, 75
bowing/whirling, 57
brainwashing, 56, 163, 235
Branch Davidian massacre, 157, 162
Brando, Marlon, 179
breathing, 80, 199–200
British Empire, 182
broken will, 40, 77, 86, 101, 208, 236
The Brothers Karamazov (Dostoyevsky), 231

Bryant, Kobe, 158
Buber, Martin, 156
Budapest String Quartet, 158
Buddha, 58
Buddhism, 106, 158

C

calling
    as blessedness, 234–235
    charitable giving vs. practicing a
        calling, 221
    clues to recognizing, 218–219
    finding of, 19, 53
    going farther afield, 220
    idea of, 210–212
    implications of discussion on,
        216–217
    Lord's work, 212–214
    mission and enablers, 217–218
    obstacles to, 214, 221–222
    overcoming obstacles, 215–216
    spiritual groups and false paths, 217
    truth about ourselves, 221–225
    victims of success, 214–215
Calvinism, 94
careers, values and, 56
caring, 154
caring empathy, 42, 191, 192
caritas, 209
Carl (case example), 12–17, 18, 20, 21,
        24, 75, 85–86, 95, 223–225
Carter, William Hodding, II, 36
case examples
    Al, 101–102, 107, 108
    Albert, 174–175
    Ben, 218
    Bernard, 158–160, 161

Carl, 12, 18, 20, 21, 24, 75, 85–
        86, 95, 223–225
Doreen, 60–62, 83–84
Doris, 96–97, 172–173, 194, 204–
        205, 206
Freddy, 175–176
Guillermo, 96
Helene, 158–160, 161
Howard, 90–91, 95, 107
Jack, 99–100, 102
Johanna, 76–77, 78, 80, 82, 213
John, 149–150, 151–152
Lance, 236–237
Lara, 75, 79
Larry, 102–103, 107
Lloyd, 187
Marlene, 109–110
Mary, 100
Max, 43–44
Michael, 175–176
Mr. Alexander, 26–27
Mr. and Mrs. Davidson, 181
Mr. B, 185
Mr. Davis, 214–216, 221
Mr. J, 212–213
Ned, 177–178
Paula, 149, 233
Penny, 202–203
Phyllis, 98, 99
Richard, 236
Sam, 172–173, 194
Sandy, 78, 205, 213, 217, 222–223
Sarah, 101, 102, 107, 217
categorical imperative, 37, 137
chanting, 57, 80, 105, 126, 128, 238
character
    calling and, 234–235
    and character disorders, 170–171

as core spiritual value, 34

defined, 168–169

as most basic spiritual quality, 169

as providing basic infrastructure of spirituality, 190

role of, 191

character armor, 162

character assessment

predictive value of, 172–173

uncertainties about, 171–172

character development

accepting responsibility, 176–177

character, defined, 168–169

character and character disorders, 170–171

cheater, 175–176

deadly sins, 180–186

Ned, the carpenter, 177–178

predictive value of character assessment, 172–173

program, 186–189

realizing potential, 178–179

refusing to be compromised, 174–175

uncertainties about character assessment, 171–172

character disorders, 59, 62, 167, 170–171

character flaws, 59, 62–63, 110, 170, 171, 184, 189

character strength, 19, 37, 49, 59, 71, 87, 171, 179, 180, 181, 182, 184, 186, 224, 227

character weaknesses, 172

charitable giving, vs. practicing a calling, 221

Chesterton, G. K., 28

Chomsky, Noam, 70

Christian Bible, 29

Christianity, 210–211, 230

Church of Synanon, 162, 165

Churchill, Winston, 117

Civilizations and Its Discontents (Freud), 118

cloud of unknowing, 148

cognitive retraining, 201, 206–207

collective unconscious, 48, 127, 243

common consciousness, 146, 147, 154

common self/common Self, 57, 131, 132, 141, 153, 168, 185, 192, 241

compartmentalization, 198, 228

compassionate empathy, ix, xii, 19, 191

compromise, refusing to be compromised, 174–175

conditioned reflexes, 63, 67, 68

conflict resolution, 97, 99, 116

conflicting values, 63, 136, 137

conscience, spiritual, 37, 62

consciousness

group consciousness, 156–157, 164

higher consciousness, 46, 57, 195, 229

intuitive consciousness, ix

parallel consciousness, 199

unitary consciousness, 156

unitive consciousness, 191, 192

unity of, 7, 147

consciousness-expanding techniques/ exercises, 128, 209

core being, 33, 48, 170, 241

core distress, assuaging of, 96–97, 98–99

core will, 186, 187

creative dissociation, 8, 198–199

creative paralysis, 83

criminal justice system
contradictory practices of, 66
rights of, 135
task of, 68
treatment of moral disorders by, 63
criminal responsibility, 137, 138, 151
critical thinking, 24, 65, 141, 142, 146, 190
The Crowd (LeBon), 117
cults
attractions and dangers of, 163–164
formation of, 161–162
overview, 162, 165–166
Curtis Institute of Music, 221
cynicism (of an indifferent world), 240–241

D

Dao, 58
Davidson, Mr. and Mrs. (case example), 181
Davis, Mr. (case example), 214–216, 221
deadly sins, 180–186
Declaration of Independence, ix, 37
The Deer Hunter (movie), 86
defensive dissociation, 198
depressed will, 72–73
depression, 17, 20, 22, 41, 42, 45, 61, 72–73, 74, 75, 79–80, 82, 83, 96, 98, 115, 165, 201, 209, 218, 221, 231
destiny
character as, 168
as other name for Spirit, 58
our creation of, 93
destructiveness, 104, 108
destrudo (death instinct), 4, 216

determinism, beyond, 69–70
deterministic causality, 69
deterministic theory, 66
diagnoses, in lay descriptive terms, 41
Diagnostic and Statistical Manual (APA), 41, 62, 115, 170
dietary rituals, 188
disenchantment, 243
disillusionment, 243
dissociated will, reparation of, 62
dissociation
creative dissociation, 8, 198–199
as defense mechanism, 89
defensive dissociation, 198
defined, 101
how it works, 85
importance of, 84
and personality disorders, 87–89
in service of health, 228
theory of, 92, 93
therapeutic dissociation, 198, 200, 201–209
dissociative mechanism, 84
dissociative reenactment, conditions of treatment for, 101–106
dissociative splitting, 53, 80, 81, 82, 87, 106. *See also* splitting
divided will, 82–84, 110, 186
divine love, as other name for Spirit, 58
do no harm, 149–150
dopamine, 76
Doreen (case example), 60–62, 83–84
Doris (case example), 96–97, 172–173, 194, 204–205, 206
Dostoyevsky, Fyodor, 231
drives, loss of control of, 182–184
drug therapy, 42
Durham Rule, 137

E

Eastern belief systems/wisdom, 196, 230
ego
    alter egos, 84, 92
    auxiliary ego, 236
    death of, 196
    defined, 48
    executive ego, 63, 82, 106
    observing ego, 62
    reparation of conscious ego, 50
Eichmann, Adolph, 139, 177
Einstein, Albert, v, 47, 48, 70, 147
élan vital (life force), 11, 127. *See also*
    life force
Ellis, Joseph, 22
empathic spirituality, 132
empathy
    caring empathy, 42, 191, 192
    channeling/interiorizing spiritual
        qualities, 208–209
    compassionate empathy, ix, xii, 19,
        191
    as core spiritual value, 34, 48
    creative dissociation, 198–199
    empathetic and cognitive
        retraining, 206–207
    exercise of as moving beyond
        ordinary consciousness, 191
    focusing attention, 199–200
    helping ordinary individuals
        reclaim spirituality,
        207–208
    loving empathy, 192
    personal spirituality, 195
    preparations for spiritual
        immersion, 200–201
    psychotic vs. spiritual, 193–195

    role of, 19
    role of in author's animosity
        towards racial persecution, 36
    sane spirituality, 196–198
    sympathetic empathy, 191
    trauma of empathic deficiency in
        parents, 204–206
    traumatic loss of in early life,
        202–203
    vulnerability of spirituality, 196
    work of therapeutic dissociation,
        201–209
empirical mind-set, 8
empirical proof, intuition vs., 138–139
enablers, mission and, 217–218
envy, 68, 127, 132, 180, 184–185, 229
Erdos, Paul, 195
Erickson, Milton, xi
Erikson, Erik, 56
Eros, 243
esprit de corps, 126, 133, 158, 193
"The Ethicist" *(New York Times*
    column), 144–145
evaluation, vs. inspiration, 25–27
evil, banality of, 139
evolution, 243
executive ego, 63, 82, 106
exercise routines, 80, 106, 188, 211
experimental controls, 25

F

faculty of intuition, 57
faith
    defined, 27
    religious faith. *See* religious faith
    replacement faiths, 241
false self, 54–55, 215, 235, 237

family admissions, in inpatient milieu therapy, 122–123

family belonging, 232

family impact, in inpatient milieu therapy, 123–125

family systems theory, 122

family therapy, 77, 122

fanatical personalities, 126

fast thinking, 139, 193

Fatal Vision (McGinniss), 88

fate, 9, 57, 58, 92, 94, 140, 209, 227, 228, 241, 243

Father Zossima (*The Brothers Karamazov*), 231

fiduciary relationship, 142

financial dealings, in therapy groups, 166

Fitzgerald, F. Scott, 83

flexibility, vs. feckless lack of character, 137

folie a deux (group-think), 187, 195

forensic psychiatry, 66

founding fathers, 37

The Founding Fathers (Ellis), 22

Frankl, Viktor, 53

Freddy (case example), 175–176

free will, 31, 64, 65–68, 70, 72, 74, 75, 79, 138, 167, 240

Free Will (Harris), 138

The Freedom of the Self (Abroms), 90, 107, 110, 149

Freud, Sigmund, x, xi, 31, 48, 49, 50, 69, 70, 83, 84, 92–93, 117–118, 128, 147, 165, 192, 202

Frieda (author's grandmother), 169

friends, 234

Fromm, Erich, 195

fundamentalisms
    cautions with, 129

literal fundamentalism, 129

political fundamentalisms, 28, 79

religious fundamentalism, 37–38, 79

scientific fundamentalism (scientism), 6, 28–31

G

Gandhi, Mahatma, 20, 30, 48, 182

Gary (case example), 4

Gates, Bill, 221

gender definition, awareness of as important for spiritual healer, 129

genuineness, 170

Gladwell, Malcolm, 139, 193, 214

global climate change, 31

gluttony, 180, 181–182, 185, 188

goals, appropriate goals, 50–51

God
    belief in, 10, 28, 199, 241
    as dead, 27
    fundamentalisms' access to mind of, 129
    happy coincidences as God acting anonymously, 7
    as higher consciousness, 46
    interpersonal, anthropomorphic God-figure, 50
    as other name for Spirit, 58, 147, 243
    personal God, 15, 239
    spiritual unconscious as, 48

Gödel's proof of incompletability of predictive knowledge, 64

gods, as other name for Spirit, 58

Goethe, v, 147

Golden Rule, 37, 135, 136

good health, 228, 234

grandchildren, importance of, 232–233

grandiosity, 69, 73, 94, 141, 184, 196,
200, 206, 222
gratitude, 12, 29, 65, 121, 134, 168,
170, 178, 184, 198, 228, 229,
233, 241, 242, 243
the great peace, 227
greed, 142, 168, 180–181
ground of being, 48, 57
group consciousness, 156–157, 164
group minds, 192, 193
group process, in outpatient therapeutic
milieu, 125–127
Group Psychology and the Analysis of the
Ego (Freud), 117
group self, 133, 192
group spirit, 14, 133, 157, 158, 164, 192
group therapy
aim of, 112
allowing members to socialize,
157–158
bad rap for, 111–112
combined with individual therapy,
106–110
hospital ward as therapeutic
milieu, 118–125
limits on socializing, 158–160
mob psychology, 117–118
personality types that can doom
aspirations of, 126, 130
psychiatric ward as microcosm,
113–116
recommended structure of,
112–113
and repair of will, 77–79
social process, 116
understanding why groups tend to
turn destructive, 116
underutilization of, 77

group will, xii, 77, 106, 109, 110, 126, 162
group-think, 195. See also folie a deux
(group-think)
guiding spirit, 13, 18–19, 21, 86, 212, 215
Guillermo (case example), 96
Gurdjieff, Georges Ivanovich, 222

H

habituation, 8, 198
Hadacol, 26–27
happiness, contrasted with blessedness,
227
Hare Krishnas, 162
harmony (with universe), 227
Harris, Sam, 138–139
healing spirit, 42
Hebrew Bible, 29
heightened awareness, 16, 57, 80, 196,
240–241
Heisenberg, Werner, 64, 69
Heisenberg's uncertainty principle, 64
Helene (case example), 158–160, 161
higher consciousness, 46, 57, 195, 229
higher power, as other name for Spirit, 58
Hinduism, 191
historical context, awareness of as
important for spiritual healer, 130
Hitler, Adolph, 22, 30, 117, 139, 147,
162, 178, 194
Holocaust, 139, 161, 164
holograms
behavioral hologram, 107, 108
as exemplars, 117, 133, 170, 199
for focusing attention, 199
as microcosms, 116, 147, 172, 187
spiritual hologram, 49
holographic patterns, 107–108

Holy Spirit, 243
hospital ward, as therapeutic milieu, 118–125
hospitalitis, 120
Howard (case example), 90–91, 95, 107
human capital, 139–141
Hume, David, 63

I

identity
    formation of, 56–57
    lost identity, 194
    race and sexuality and, 55
    as spiritual term, 51
    true self and, 53
identity formation, awareness of as important for spiritual healer, 129–130
illusions, and moral conflicts, 141
impulsivity, 74, 75
In the Belly of the Beast (Abbott), 137
inborn genetic structure, 243
incompletability of predictive knowledge, 64, 70
indeterminism, 70
individual psychodynamic therapy
    combined with group therapy, 106–110
    overselling of, 77
individual rights, conflicts with social order, 136–138
individual will, subjugation of, 162
influential spirituality, 69
information
    compared to wisdom, 148
    as mechanism of setting limits, 104
inpatient milieu therapy, 125

insanity defense, 137
insensitivities, 61, 107, 207, 208
inspiration, 21, 25–27, 29, 34, 36, 52, 57, 71, 112, 115, 132, 172, 185, 242
instinctual repression, 93
integrity
    its loss and repair, 235–238
    moral integrity, 38, 39, 55, 143, 150
    as spiritual term, 51
internal saboteur, 14, 16, 54, 59, 61, 80, 82, 85, 87, 88–89, 90, 92, 95–97, 100, 103, 105, 106, 108, 110, 168, 172, 186, 187, 198, 202, 205
interview, initial clinical, 40–42
intrinsic spiritual potential, 208
intuition
    contamination of, 141
    defined, 19
    vs. empirical proof, 138–139
    faculty of intuition, 57
    as fallible, 24, 141
    as moral base of choice, 30
    moral intuition, 39, 62, 139
    refined by critical thinking, 142, 239
intuitive awareness, 9, 148, 211
intuitive consciousness, ix
intuitive knowledge, 9, 148
intuitive moral truth, ix

J

J., Mr. (case example), 212–213
Jack (case example), 99–100, 102
Jackson, Phil, 158
James, William, x
Jane (case example), 2–3, 5, 6
Janet, Pierre, 84, 92

Jefferson, Thomas, 37, 48

Jesus, 33, 210

jogging, 188

Johanna (case example), 76–77, 78, 80, 82, 213

John (case example), 149–150, 151

Johnson, Lyndon, 37

Jones, Maxwell, 118

Jonestown tragedy, 117, 161, 162

Judaism, 169, 180, 201, 230

Jung, Carl, 6, 48, 49, 127, 165

K

Kafka, Franz, 244

Kahneman, Daniel, 139, 193

Kammerer, Paul, 7

Kant, Immanuel, x, 33, 138, 142, 147, 237

Khosla, Vinod, 215

King, Martin Luther, Jr., 36, 48, 178, 179

knowledge

    compared to wisdom, 148

    incompletability of predictive knowledge, 64, 70

    intuitive knowledge, 9, 148

    scientific knowledge, 24, 30, 31, 64, 69, 129, 240

    spiritual knowledge, 9–11, 24, 69

Kohut, Heinz, 56, 206

Koresh, David, 157

Korngold, Erich, 179–180

L

Lamictal (lamotrigine), 76

Lance (case example), 236–237

Lara (case example), 75, 79

Larry (case example), 102–103, 107

leaders, personal qualities of, 127–128

LeBon, Gustave, 117, 164, 192

Levenkron, Steven, 3

life force, 11, 18, 46, 57, 58, 147, 155, 178, 220, 228, 231. *See also élan vital* (life force)

life mission, 217

lifework, 212, 215, 220

limits, setting of, 103–106, 146

Lincoln, Abraham, 20, 30, 37, 48, 57, 178

living hell, state of, 231

Lloyd (case example), 187

Locke, John, 63

logical positivism, 28

Lord's work, 212–214

Los Angeles Lakers, 157

losses, making good on, 153–154

lost identity, 194

love

    divine love, as other name for Spirit, 58

    platonic spiritual love, 229–231

    spiritual love, 132, 202, 229–231

    tough love, 154, 178, 189

love bonds, spiritual bonds as, 132

love partners, 229, 230

lovemaking, 182

loving empathy, 192

Lula (author's childhood cook), 169

lust, 180, 182–183

M

Madoff, Bernard, 89, 161

Mailer, Norman, 136–137

Maimonides, Moses, v, 29, 33, 34, 171

Mandela, Nelson, 30, 48, 57

Mann, Thomas, v, 92, 147

Mao Zedong, 194

marital bond, spiritualizing of, 157

Marlene (case example), 109–110

marriage, as spiritual phenomenon, 91

martial arts, 81, 97, 105, 140, 209

Mary (case example), 100

Maslow, Abraham, x

mass murder, 37, 93, 117, 134, 161, 176

Massachusetts Mental Health Center, x

Max (case example), 43–44

McDonald, Jeffrey, 87–88

McGinniss, Joe, 88

McNabb, Donovan, 157

Mead, George Herbert, 231

meaningful coincidences, 5, 6, 7

medications

    in case of Johanna, 76

    as lesser form of treatment, 32

    as mechanism of setting limits,
        104, 105

    as only one among many
        approaches, 42

meditation, 17, 21, 35, 42, 50, 57, 80,
    99, 105, 126, 128, 140, 198,
    199, 209, 238, 240

mental health

    emphasis on, 58

    spirituality and, 52–53

mentoring/mentors, 11, 52, 61, 62, 80,
    128, 170, 175, 213, 216, 217,
    222, 229, 237, 242

Michael (case example), 175–176

milieu therapy, 111, 118, 119, 125

Mind-Spirit-Will, 147

mission, and enablers, 217–218

mob psychology, 117–118

mode of evaluation, 25

mode of inspiration, 25–27

Mogel, Wendy, 30

mood disorders, 75, 79, 105, 106, 193,
    201, 207

mood stabilizers, 75, 76, 86, 105

Moonies, 162

moral awareness, 147

moral code

    advocacy and what it entails, 146

    attractions and dangers of cults,
        163–164

    breaking conventional therapy
        rule, 157–158

    cautionary tale of Helene and
        Bernard, 158–160

    conflicts between individual rights
        and social order, 136–137

    critical thinking, 142

    cult formation, 161–162

    cults, 162

    do no harm, 149–150

    enhancers of human capital,
        139–140

    group consciousness, 156–157

    human capital and spiritual values,
        140–141

    illusions and moral conflicts, 141

    implications of moral-spiritual
        truth, 146–149

    intuition vs. empirical proof,
        138–139

    issue of making amends, 149

    limits on socializing, 158–160

    main terms of modern humanistic
        and spiritual moral code,
        143–144

    making good on losses, 153–154

morality and anomalous position
of psychotherapy, 142–146
overview, 134–136
possibility of lesser amends,
152–153
rules of spiritual group, 166–167
spiritual dimension of outpatient
milieu, 155–156
for therapy, 154–155
treatment philosophy, 164–166
treatment when amends cannot be
made, 151–152
moral conflicts, illusions and, 141
moral disorders, forms of, 63
moral exception, 147
moral insanity, 161, 176
moral integrity, 38, 39, 55, 143, 150
moral intuition, 39, 62, 139
moral leveling, 178
moral neutrality, 11, 61, 142, 150, 170
moral rehabilitation, 136
moral relativism, 142, 241
moral treatment, 39, 63, 170, 207
morality, and anomalous position of
psychotherapy, 142–146
moral-spiritual truth, implications of,
146–149
Morgan, Juliette, 36
morphogenic fields, 71
Moses (biblical), 33
Mozart, Wolfgang Amadeus, 37, 147,
180
Mr. Sammler's Planet (Bellow), 148
multiple personality disorder (MPD),
84, 91–92
mutism, 72
My Stroke of Insight (Taylor), 7

N

narcissism, 54, 69, 71–72, 79, 141, 147,
163, 200, 204, 221
narcissistic injury, 69
Nazis, 28, 55, 56, 148, 153, 180, 213
NBA, 23
Ned (case example), 177–178
neurotransmitters, 76
new spiritual age, 46
New York Times, 144
nickel-and-dime mishaps, 152
nickel-and-dime morality, 146
Nietzsche, Friedrich, 27, 154, 180
nihilism, 26, 33, 242
nocebo effect, 26
nondirective therapy, 51, 104
norepinephrine, 76

O

obesity, 168, 181, 188
observers, introduction of into patient's
life, 101–103, 106–107
observing ego, 62
obsessive-compulsive personalities, 42,
50, 96, 126, 130
obstructed will, 81, 83. *See also* blocked
will
O'Neal, Shaquille, 157–158
one-mindedness, 140
operant conditioning, 63, 68
oppositionalism, 74, 187
organized religion, as structured
activity, 105
organizing principle, as other name for
Spirit, 58
Orgone Box therapy, 162

Orthogenic School, 222

outpatient therapeutic milieu
  group process in, 125–127
  spiritual dimension of, 155–156

overeating, 181

Owens, Terrell, 157

P

Palestinians, 182

paradigm shift, 22, 64

parallel consciousness, 199

paralytic inertia, 78

paranoid belligerence, 75

paranoid personalities, 126, 130, 131,
  156, 230

paranormal powers, 22

parapsychologists, 192

parental alienation syndromes, 56

Parfit, Derek, x, 33

parsimony, principle of, 8

passionate knowing, 209

passivity, 74, 115, 185–186

Patriot Act, 136

Paula (case example), 149, 233

Penny (case example), 202

personal sanctions, as mechanism of
  setting limits, 104–105

personal spirituality, 195

personality, integrating conflicting
  parts of, 238–240

personality disorders
  addictive disorders/personalities,
    77, 110, 126, 130, 230
  antisocial personalities, 39, 126,
    130–131, 140, 161, 230
  borderline personalities, 104, 113,
    114, 126, 154, 197

character disorders reduced to, 62

dissociation and, 87–89

fanatical personalities, 126

multiple personality disorder
  (MPD), 84, 91–92

obsessive-compulsive personalities,
  42, 50, 96, 126, 130

paranoid personalities, 126, 130,
  131, 156, 230

pessimism hovering over treatment
  of, 98

psychopathic personalities, 89,
  130–131

self-defeating personality patterns,
  41, 42, 52, 62, 87, 93–95,
  101, 103, 112, 115

sociopathic personalities, 116, 126,
  130–131, 156

split personality, 84

split-off subpersonality, 16

subpersonalities, 16, 85, 87, 88, 91,
  92, 97

personality theory, 93

Philadelphia Eagles, 157

philanthropic giving, 221

phobic anxiety, 61, 74

Phyllis (case example), 98, 99

placebo effect, xii, 25, 115

Plato, 8, 9, 10, 198

platonic spiritual love, 229–231

play, 211

Pol Pot, 147

political fundamentalisms, 28, 79

Ponzi schemes, 89, 161

positive beliefs, making transition to, 10

post-traumatic stress disorder (PTSD),
  85, 86, 89

potential, realization of, 178–179

prayer, 17, 21, 27, 35, 42, 50, 57, 80, 81, 105, 128, 140, 198, 239, 240
primal raging, 183
primary process thinking, 193, 194, 196
principle(s)
  acausal connecting principle, 6
  anthropic principle, 242
  Heisenberg's uncertainty principle, 64
  organizing principle, as other name for Spirit, 58
  principle of parsimony, 8
  universal moral principles, 139, 156, 191
productive rituals, 105
prophetic dreams, 21
pseudo-communities, 79, 166
psyche, anatomy of, 48–50
psychiatric ward, as microcosm, 113–116
psychiatry, author's early experience in, 1–3, 5
psychic determinism, theory of, 31–32, 63
psychic glue, 197
psychological growth, 43–44, 45, 159
psychologism, 28, 31–33
psychomotor retardation, 72
psychopathic personalities, 89, 130–131
psychotherapeutic change, theory of, 24
psychotherapy
  defined, 24, 33
  on moral truths, 142
  role of, 63
psychotic, vs. spiritual, 193–195
PTSD (post-traumatic stress disorder), 85, 86, 89
purpose (of life), 19, 51

Q

quantum physics, 65, 66, 69, 156

R

race, sexuality and identity and, 55
Rachmaninov, Sergei, 83
racism, author's experience of, 35–39
radical Islamism, 164
rage, 85, 123, 155, 180, 183–184, 187, 202
Rajneesh, Bhagwan Shree, 117, 157, 190–191
Rank, Otto, 53, 165, 206
Raper, Arthur F., 36
rational belief system, 163
Rawls, John, x, 33
reading the tea leaves, 217
reality
  Spirit, as ultimate reality, 10
  spiritual reality, ix, x, 8, 15, 23, 200
redemption, 151, 211
reenactment, 90–91, 101–106
regression, passivity and, 185–186
Reich, Wilhelm, 162
relative values, 241
relativity, 178
religious faith, 10, 23, 27, 28, 29, 31, 46, 97, 241
religious fundamentalism, 37–38, 79
replacement faiths, 28
repressed instinctual pressures, 70
repression, theory of, 92
responsibility, acceptance of, 176–177
Richard (case example), 236
Robinson, Sugar Ray, 97
Rogers, Carl, 104

Roosevelt, Franklin D., 179

Rossini, Gioacchino, 83

rules

Durham Rule, 137

Golden Rule, 37, 135, 136

of spiritual group, 166–167

S

Sakharov, Andrei, 30, 48, 57

Salem, 164

Sam (case example), 172–173, 194

sanctions, as mechanism of setting
limits, 104–105

Sandusky, Jerry, 138

Sandy (case example), 78, 205, 213,
217, 222–223

sane spirituality, 196–198

Sarah (case example), 101, 102, 107,
217

schadenfreude, 6, 127, 208, 230

Schopenhauer, Arthur, 92, 93

Schrödinger, Erwin, 69

Schwartz, Morris, 119

science

as misconceived, 63–65

role of, 51

scientific empiricism, 8–9

scientific fundamentalism (scientism),
6, 28–31

scientific knowledge, 24, 30, 31, 64, 69,
129, 240

scientific mind-set, 5, 6–7

scientism, 6, 28–31

Scientologists, 162

Self, xiii, 46, 48, 49, 50, 51, 91, 97, 99,
141, 147, 153, 156, 171, 209,
212, 227, 244

self psychologists, 56

self-consciousness, 49, 211

self-defeating personality patterns, 41,
42, 52, 62, 87, 93–95, 101, 103,
112, 115

self-denial, 182

self-deprivation, 182

self-destructive instinct (*destrudo*), 216

self-development (of spiritual healers),
128

self-discipline, 180

selfs

common self/common Self. *See*
common self/common Self

false self, 54–55, 215, 235, 237

group self, 133, 192

Self. *See* Self

true self. *See* true self

universal Self, Mind, or Will, 48, 58

self-serving rationalizations, 95

Self-Will/self-will, 70, 85, 86, 134

Semrad, Elvin, xi

serendipity, 5–8, 93

serotonin, 76

sexual liaisons, in therapy groups, 157,
166

sexuality, race and identity and, 55

"shall do" values, 241

"shall not" values, 241

shattered will, 84–85

Sheldrake, Rupert, 71

Sibelius, Jean, 83

significant play, 211

sins, deadly, 180–186

sixth sense, 57

Skinner, B. F., 68

sloth, 180, 185–186

SNRIs, 76

social conditioning, 37, 137, 141

social order, conflicts with individual
    rights, 136–138

social process, 115, 116

socializing outside group, xii, 103, 111,
    158, 159–160, 166

sociopathic personalities, 116, 126,
    130–131, 156

Socrates, xiii, 33

Solzhenitsyn, Aleksandr, 30

Soul, defined, 10

soul mates, 229, 230

Spirit
    access to, 80
    defined, ix, 7, 10, 49, 240
    fundamental truths of, 156
    as higher consciousness, 46
    as neither hostile nor indifferent to
        human enterprise, 240
    other names for, 57–58
    spontaneous encounters with, 57
    as ultimate reality, 10
    unification with, 48

spirit, love and creation/destruction of,
    231

spiritual, psychotic vs., 193–195

spiritual aggregation, 118

spiritual awareness
    achievement of, 80, 155-156
    and exercise of empathy, 191
    gaining of, 7
    growth in as finding way through
        cloud of unknowing, 148
    as needing to be integrated into
        everyday worldview, 200
    outpatient milieu as providing
        conditions for
    practices for reaching realm of, 140

Revelation as, 9

role of, 38, 196

as substitute for religious faith, 23

spiritual bonds, formation of, 132–133

spiritual care group, 79

spiritual conscience, 37, 62

spiritual crisis, 45–46

spiritual depths, 70

spiritual framework, 7, 12–17, 20, 81, 89

spiritual group
    animosities in, 158
    benefits of effective spiritual group
        therapy, 155, 156, 215, 216
    changing psychological group into,
        113
    contrasted with cult, 166
    defined, 132
    and false paths, 217
    formation/development of, 34
    information conveyed by, 222
    marriage as, 91
    personal qualities of leader of,
        127–128
    preconditions for formation of,
        130, 131, 229–230
    rules of, 166–167

spiritual growth, 17, 44, 52, 81, 106,
    125, 130, 147, 154, 158, 170,
    171, 184

spiritual guidance, 17–19, 33–34, 51

spiritual healer, education of, 128

spiritual hologram, 49

spiritual immersion, preparations for,
    200–201

spiritual knowledge
    according to Freud, 69
    consequences of for therapy, 11
    introduction to, 9–11

as part of superstructure, 24

spiritual life, hallmarks of, 47–48

spiritual love, 132, 202, 229–231

spiritual phenomenon, marriage as, 91

spiritual practices, 80–81, 105, 240

spiritual qualities, channeling and
    interiorizing of, 208–209

spiritual reality, ix, x, 8, 15, 23, 200

spiritual support, group therapy as
    source of, 108–109

spiritual terms, 18, 51, 56, 236

spiritual therapy
    goal of, 199, 208
    as humane therapy, 39–40
    as integrative and corrective,
        20–21
    as presupposing acts of
        transcendence, 65
    ultimate purpose of, 227

spiritual truth, 8, 9, 10, 28–31, 34, 51,
    128, 201, 211

spiritual unconscious, xi, 48–49

spiritual unity, 110, 240

spiritual vacuum, 163

spiritual values, 140–141, 143, 230

spirituality
    attainment of, 57–58
    character as providing basic
        infrastructure of, 190
    decontamination of, 50
    empathic spirituality, 132
    essence of, 131
    helping ordinary individuals
        reclaim, 207–208
    influential spirituality, 69
    and mental health, 52–53
    in modern terms, 46–47
    personal spirituality, 195

sane spirituality, 196–198
    vulnerability of, 196

Spirit-Will, 110, 141

split awareness, 200

split personality, 83, 84

split will, 83, 85–86

split-off awareness, 205

split-off memory, 150

split-off partial selves, 88, 90, 209

split-off saboteur, 54, 59, 61, 85, 88,
    106, 172, 204, 206, 232

split-off subpersonality, 16

split-off tormentor, 203

splitting, xii, 53, 54, 80, 82, 85, 86,
    87, 89–90, 91, 96, 101, 108,
    116, 198, 202, 205. *See also*
    dissociative splitting

SSRIs, 76

Stalin, Joseph, 22, 161, 178

Stanton, Alfred, 118

string theory, 64

structured activity, as mechanism of
    setting limits, 104, 105

sublimation, x

subpersonalities, 16, 85, 87, 88, 91, 92,
    97

Sufism, 57, 227

suicide, 45, 86, 87, 88, 117, 135, 155,
    162, 183

Sullivan, J. W. N., 72

supra-individual forces, 71

suprapersonal awareness, 50

supra-temporal agency, 70

survival mechanisms, 148

swimming, 188

Sybil (Schreiber), 91

sympathetic empathy, 191

symptom relief, 42–43, 44, 45, 154

Synanon, Church of, 162, 165
synchronicity, 5–8, 90

T

Talmud, 29, 30, 210
Taylor, Jill Bolte, 7
tea leaves, reading of, 217
Teilhard de Chardin, Pierre, 11, 240
theories
    deterministic theory, 66
    family systems theory, 122
    personality theory, 93
    string theory, 64
    theory of dissociation, 92, 93
    theory of psychic determinism,
        31–32, 63
    theory of psychotherapeutic
        change, 24
    theory of repression, 92
therapeutic cult, defined, 163
therapeutic dissociation, 198, 200,
    201–209
therapy, moral code for, 154–155
Thorazine, 32
thought disorders, 41, 75, 79, 105, 106,
    201, 207, 209
thought-broadcasting, 192
The Three Faces of Eve (Thigpen and
    Cleckley), 91
tikkun olam (Hebrew for repairing the
    world), 15, 16
Tofranil, 32
tolerance, vs. dogmatic belief, 137
Torah, 201, 210
tough love, 154, 178, 189
transference resolution, 236
trauma, types of, 86–87

treatment
    barriers to, 98–99
    medications as lesser form of, 32
    moral treatment, 39, 63, 170, 207
    philosophy of, 164–166
    when amends cannot be made,
        151–152
true moral therapy, 52
true self, xii, 15, 17, 18, 24, 33, 34, 50,
    53, 54, 56, 58, 62, 96, 148, 211,
    212, 215, 216, 227, 234, 235,
    237, 241, 244
true spiritual self, gaining access to, 49
tunnel vision, 243
Twain, Mark, 147
twelve-step programs, 98, 110,
    130, 149. *See also* Alcoholics
    Anonymous (AA)

U

unacceptable notions, 21–24
uncertainty principle (Heisenberg), 64
unconscious
    collective unconscious, 48, 127, 243
    spiritual unconscious, xi, 48–49
unconscious motivation, 31, 69, 71
unconscious repressed, xi, 49
unique mission, 211
unitary consciousness, 156
unitive consciousness, 191, 192
universal moral code, 134–135
universal moral principles, 139, 156, 191
universal Self, Mind, or Will, 48, 58
universal will, 10, 19
University of Wisconsin Hospitals
    (Madison), 119
unknowing, cloud of, 148

unpredictability, 70
Upanishads, 156

V

value assumptions, 22, 23, 31
value change, x, 38, 45, 52, 143
value-free nondirection, compared to
    value-directed prescriptions,
    78–79
value(s)
    absolute values, 179, 241–242
    and careers, 56
    conflicting values, 63, 136, 137
    relative values, 241
    "shall do" values, 241
    "shall not" values, 241
    as spiritual term, 51
    spiritual values, 140–141, 143, 230
visualization, 50, 57, 80, 105, 126, 240
vocation, 210–212. *See also* calling

W

Waco tragedy, 117, 157, 162
walking, 188
Weiss, Edoardo, 4
Welles, Orson, 179
Western worldview/culture/moral code,
    29, 71, 117, 129, 181, 196, 201,
    230
Whitaker, Carl, xi, 122
Wilkomirski, B., 54
will
    anchoring of, 187–189
    auxiliary will, 236
    blockage of, 60–62, 73, 75, 77, 80.
        See also blocked will

bound will, 72, 75
broken will, 40, 77, 86, 101, 208,
    236
core will, 186, 187
defined, 65
depressed will, 72–73
development of, 73–74
divided will. *See* divided will
free will. *See* free will
group repair of, 77–78
group will, 77, 106, 109, 110, 126,
    162
    as not respectable subject for
        discussion among scientific
        elite, 63
    obstructed will, 81, 83. *See also*
        blocked will
    as outside materialistic causal
        chains, 64
    paralysis and activation of, 59–81
    pathologies of, 74–76
    shattered will, 84–85
    as spiritual term, 51
    split will, 83, 85–86
    universal will, 10, 19
    weakness of, 155
will to death, 4
will to health, 1, 3–4, 18, 40, 42, 58,
    75, 81, 86, 113, 146, 186, 207
will to life, 58, 73, 155
William of Occam, 8, 9, 10, 28, 63, 193
wisdom
    of the ages, 225–226
    benefits of acquiring, 156
    Eastern belief systems/wisdom,
        196, 230
    information/knowledge as
        compared to, 148

spiritual awareness as necessary
    precondition of gaining, 148
Wittgenstein, Ludwig, 47, 49
work therapy, 120–121
world soul, 80, 127
world spirit, 231

Y

yoga, 17, 50, 57, 80, 81, 105, 140, 201,
    209
You Are Not Your Illness (Topf), 228

Z

Zohar, 29